Your Child's Symptoms Explained

David Haslam has been a General Practitioner since 1976. He writes and broadcasts regularly on medical topics and is a frequent contributor to *Practical Parenting*. He is the author of eight books, and is Vice Chairman of the General Practitioner Writers Association. He is a Patron of Serene (formerly Cry-Sis) – alongside Jane Asher and Claire Rayner – a judge for the Parent Friendly Awards and a member of the Huggies Childcare Panel, as well as being Chairman of the Examination Board for the Royal College of General Practitioners.

Dr Haslam is married with two children and lives in East Anglia. His special interests are music and photography.

Also by David Haslam

Sleepless Children
Travelling with Children
ParentStress
Mothercare Guide for
the Expectant Father
Bulimia: a guide for
sufferers and their families*
Food Fights:
a practical guide for parents worried about
their children's eating habits*
Coping with a Termination:
advice on the emotional and practical difficulties
of an unwanted pregnancy*

* available from Vermilion – to order copies of
these three titles call TBS DIRECT on 01621 819596
(p & p free).

Dr David Haslam

Your Child's Symptoms Explained

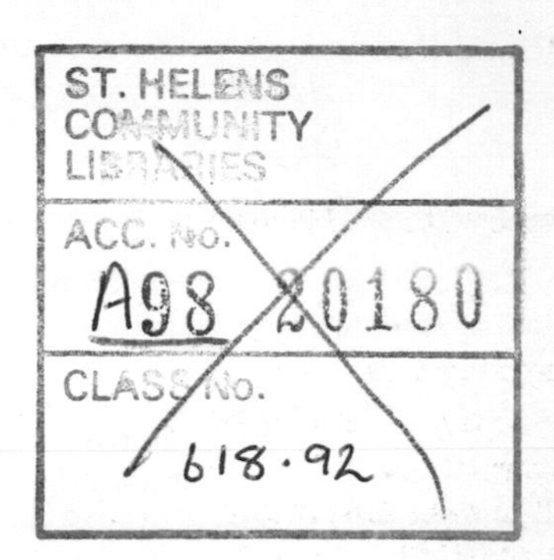

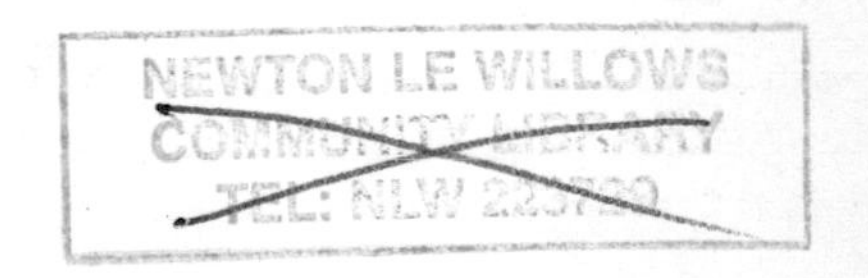

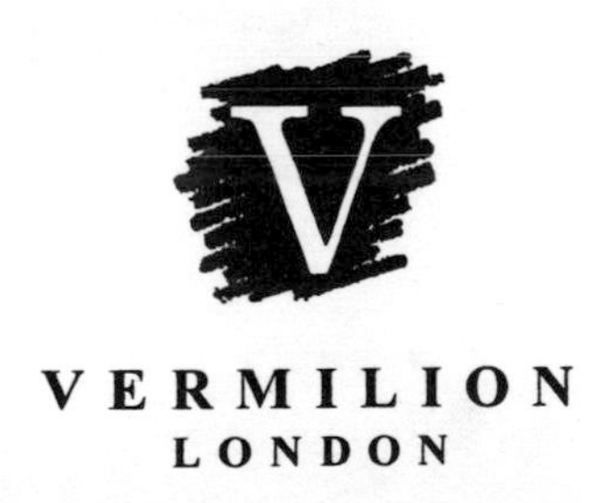

VERMILION
LONDON

1 3 5 7 9 10 8 6 4 2

First published in the United Kingdom in 1997 by Vermilion, an imprint of Ebury Press
Random House UK Ltd
Random House, 20 Vauxhall Bridge Road, SW1V 2SA

Random House Australia (Pty) Limited
20 Alfred Street, Milsons Point, Sydney,
New South Wales 2061, Australia

Random House New Zealand Limited
18 Poland Road, Glanfield
Auckland 10, New Zealand

Random House South Africa (Pty) Limited
Endulini, 5a Jubilee Road,
Park Town 2193, South Africa

Random House UK Limited Reg No 954009

A CIP catalogue record for this title is available from the British Library

ISBN: 0 74 932289 6

Typeset by Avon Dataset Ltd, Bidford on Avon, Warks
Printed and bound in Great Britain
by Cox & Wyman Ltd, Reading, Berkshire

Papers used by Vermilion are natural, recyclable products made from wood grown in sustainable forests.

For my daughter Katy
and my son Chris

Please note

Whilst the author has endeavoured to ensure that this book is entirely accurate and up-to-date, it can never be possible in a book of this nature to cover every conceivable eventuality with any given child. For this reason, the author would strongly urge the reader to seek individual medical advice whenever possible. Neither the author nor the publishers can be held liable for any errors or omissions, or for any action that might be taken as a consequence of following the advice in the book.

Contents

Introduction 1

1 **How to use this book** 5

2 **When to call a doctor** 9

3 **Childhood Symptoms** 19
The child with a fever 21
The child who is in pain 27
The child who is crying 32
The child with a cough 39
The child who wheezes 51
The child with a cold 61
The child with a sore throat 68
The child with earache 73
The child with a discharging ear 82
The child with hearing problems 85
The child with a stiff, painful or swollen neck 92
The child with a headache 96
The child with nose problems 105
The child with mouth problems 112
The child with toothache 116
The child who vomits 120
The child with diarrhoea 126
The child with constipation 134
The child with abnormal stools 140
The child with abdominal pains 147
The child with problems passing urine 155
The child with problems with the genitals or groin 171
The child with an itch 182
The child with a rash 189

The child with nappy rash 231
The child with a verruca or wart 235
The child with allergies 238
The child with red eyes 260
The child with other eye problems 269
The child who has a fit 274
The child with bone or joint problems 283

4 **Infectious Diseases** 295

5 **A Guide to Children's Medicines** 299
Giving medicines to children 319
A home medicine chest 323

6 **Practical Techniques** 327
How to take your child's temperature 329
Emergency resuscitation for parents 330

7 **Useful Organisations** 333

Index of symptoms 337
Index 339

Acknowledgements

This book is based on over twenty years' experience in general practice, and is largely based on my observations of the large number of parents and children who have consulted me. I owe a great debt of gratitude to all of them, but I also sought specific advice in a number of areas. The chart giving brief details of all the main infectious illnesses is adapted from a chart developed by Dr John R. Bailey, Consultant in Communicable Disease Control, for the East Norfolk Health Commission, and is reproduced with his very kind permission, and also the kind consent of the copyright holders, the Specialist Health Promotion Services, at the James Paget Hospital NHS Trust in Great Yarmouth.

The section on 'A Guide to Children's Medicines' is based on an article that I originally wrote for *Practical Parenting* and is included here with the kind permission of the editor. I would also like to thank Carole Blake and Victoria Hipps, without whom this entire project would not have been possible, and also Cherry Toyer for her secretarial help.

Finally, despite the training I received at medical school, I learnt more about childcare from my wife, Barbara, and my children, Katy and Chris, than I could ever have gained from all the books in the world. If this book does show any understanding of what it can feel like to be a worried parent, then that is because I, too, have been a worried parent! I cannot thank my family enough.

Introduction

Every parent worries about their child becoming ill. Take it from me – it's no easier when you are a doctor. Your own children are so very precious that it can be remarkably difficult working out how best to treat them, when to seek help, and what medicines you might use.

Before we become parents, we really don't know what to expect. None of us can ever be sufficiently prepared. When our first child arrives, it can sometimes seem as if we are instantly expected to become experts in diagnosis and treatment. Tiny babies seem so dreadfully frail, and new parents are bound to feel worried and concerned, and worried about being over-concerned. It seems so difficult to get the balance right. After all, how do you know whether you are being too anxious about each and every sniffle and cough, or whether you are ignoring dangerous symptoms that might be the start of meningitis or something even worse?

If you go to the surgery about an illness which turns out to be trivial, please don't feel embarrassed or think that you've wasted the doctor's time. If you consult a doctor because you are worried and leave with the worry taken away, then how can that possibly have been a waste of anybody's time? Indeed, one of a family doctor's most important roles should be teaching parents about what is normal, what is not, and how best the parents can usually deal with their child. If you don't leave the doctor's with a prescription, but instead have had a helpful and positive discussion about how to cope with this sort of problem in future, then the consultation will have been worthwhile. Parents are, without a shadow of a doubt, the most important people in any medical care system for any child. However good your G.P., your practice nurse, or your health visitor, you are the one who knows your child best, and you are the one who needs to know when to get the professionals involved. I remember seeing a child with meningitis some years ago who very nearly died, but whose life was not saved by me and the antibiotics that I gave, nor by the hospital paediatricians who were brilliant throughout, or even the team on the intensive care unit where the child spent three terrifyingly unconscious days. The child's life was actually saved by his mother. It was she who telephoned me and described what was happening in a way that meant that the whole of the emergency team could get into action straight away. Experts are no use at all if parents do not seek help from them in time, and equally they will not be able to cope if every parent presents every single symptom. Parents make all the difference to any effective childcare system.

When I first became a junior hospital doctor in a nationally respected specialist children's hospital, my consultant – a highly respected and brilliant man called Ben Wood – took me to one side. 'I will think I've done a good job with you,' he said, 'if at the end of six months here you are able to recognise when a child is ill and when it is not.' To begin with I thought he was teasing me, and making fun of my inexperience. But he was absolutely right. It can be extremely difficult to pick up the warning signs of some conditions, or differentiate with confidence between something minor and something serious.

And of course, if deciding when a child is ill can be difficult for doctors, then it can be even harder for parents. There are always going to be occasions when you simply cannot be sure, and those are usually the occasions when you should consult a doctor. You are the expert in your own child, but your doctor should have the experience of dealing with countless other children and the two of you together should make a good team.

Many other childcare books expect you to know the diagnosis of what is wrong with your child, so that you can look the problem up in the index. That is fine if you know that your child has asthma, or tonsillitis, or some other clear-cut problem, but it is little help if you have no real idea what is happening.

That is where this book will help you. The chapters are arranged by symptoms. If your child has a sore throat, you will simply look up that chapter and then be guided through all the various possible diagnoses and treatments. If your child has a headache, I will look at all the likely causes and what you can do about them. And if you are sure what the diagnosis is, possibly after visiting the doctor, the indexing system will allow you to gain more information readily and speedily.

More than anything, I want to help you answer many of those questions that parents find themselves asking – what should I feed my child if he or she has a tummy upset? Why does my daughter always cough at night? What medicines should I keep in the house? This book will concentrate on the common conditions of childhood. I won't be dealing with the real rarities, but instead will concentrate on those day-to-day conditions that cause parents the most concern.

An equally important function of this book is to provide detailed information for you to read after you have seen the doctor. Most doctors are extremely busy, and simply don't have the time to give as detailed an explanation as they might like. Nevertheless I always find it terribly sad when I see a child who has maybe had four or five ear infections, and I suddenly realise the parents know nothing whatsoever about ear infections except that they hurt and the yellow medicine takes the pain away. This book can function as an additional source of information to that provided by your doctor, though do remember that every child is different and that you and your doctor are the experts on your child. And – if in doubt, ask.

No one can ever promise you that parenthood is easy, but having clear information at your fingertips can make all the difference to how confident you feel. In years gone by, most young parents had their own parents living nearby. There was always someone to turn to for advice, someone who had seen it all before. In most Western countries the days of this close-knit extended family have long gone. Young parents often have no one to turn to when they are puzzled or concerned – no one other than doctors, health visitors, or other healthcare professionals. If grandparents do live nearby, they are unlikely to be grandparents as pictured in most traditional children's books – sitting in a rocking chair, whilst the smell of home-baked bread wafts in from the kitchen. Today's grandparents are frequently still active in their work, out at aerobics classes, or enjoying a highly active retirement. The world has moved on, and young parents can often feel abandoned. That is where this book can begin to help you. It will unravel the serious from the minor, and point you in the right direction when it comes to knowing how to care for your child. I really do hope that you find this book useful. Parents need all the help they can get.

Section One

How to use this book

The purpose of this book is to act as a guide to the commonest symptoms that affect children. It concentrates on infants (babies in their first year) and children aged up to twelve, and whilst it cannot aim to be a complete textbook of child health, it will allow you to understand what may be wrong with your child and how best you can help. You may even use it in conjunction with some of the other encyclopaedic childcare books that can give vast amounts of information, but are far less helpful in unravelling a crisis. This book is a handbook. Keep it to hand!

The book is arranged very simply. The main chapters all refer to specific problems, and these will be self-explanatory. As an example, chapter headings include:

The child who vomits
The child with diarrhoea
The child with constipation
The child with abdominal pain

If your child has any of the common childhood medical symptoms then you should simply look up the relevant chapter. The chapter will describe all the commonest causes of this particular symptom, how you might try to tell them apart, which ones are serious, how they should be treated, and so on.

If you are less certain about what is causing the problem, then turn to the index. The index will guide you to the part, or parts, of the book that deal with this particular problem or symptom.

In addition, the book will guide you clearly when you need to refer to a passage elsewhere in the text. To take a simple example, one of the commonest causes of abdominal pain in children is a condition called mesenteric adenitis. Mesenteric adenitis typically follows a throat infection. Everyone knows that the glands in the neck can swell up with a sore throat. Not everyone realises that glands in the abdomen can swell up in the same way and cause a tummy ache that can be easily confused with appendicitis. Once I have explained how this happens, it would not be logical to give a full explanation of throat infections in the middle of the chapter on abdominal pain, so the text will simply refer you to the relevant page in the relevant chapter.

There is also a clear section on when you should call a doctor, as well as an appendix which describes the medication you should keep in a simple home medicine chest. You may be surprised how few drugs are listed here. The simple fact is that the vast majority of drugs that are on sale for use in childhood are superfluous. Many parents believe that they should have linctuses, laxatives, vitamins, and virtually a miniature chemist's shop in their bathroom cupboard. This isn't necessary. A few simple things are all you need.

More than anything else it is vital to remember that whilst this book will often give you all the information that you need, there will be situations where you will still be in doubt. If you are in doubt, do contact a doctor. It is always better to be safe than sorry.

Section Two

When to call a doctor

Sick children can be a very real worry. Whilst this book should be a very real help on those occasions when you are concerned, and whilst very many minor conditions can certainly be treated at home, nevertheless if you are worried then you really should seek advice. Do this if you aren't certain what is wrong, or if what you thought was a minor problem takes longer than usual to clear up. Throughout the book I will be giving clear guidelines at to when you do need medical help, but I cannot be there with you and your child. It makes far more sense to be safe than sorry.

Although the individual sections of this book will give specific guidance for specific problems, it is none the less still possible to make some very general rules about when you should seek medical help or advice, and these are summarised in table one. Perhaps more than anything, you need to take into account your child's age. In general, the younger the child the more potentially serious could any infection be, and at any age you can be reassured if your child is eating well and seems normally energetic.

With small babies it is particularly difficult to make any foolproof, hard and fast rules about when you should call a doctor. With a first baby in particular it is probably wise to err on the side of caution. Most experienced doctors would be the first to recognise that the true expert in any particular child is that child's parent. If you are concerned, then the doctor should at the very least make some assessment of the situation until he or she can put your mind at rest.

Very frequently, of course, there may not be any real need

to see the doctor. This is particularly the case if your child has an illness like chickenpox, there is an epidemic in your area, and you feel certain about the diagnosis. However, there cannot be any hard and fast rules about how long you should wait before getting help. If in doubt, ask. Most general practices are these days becoming more and more available for consultation by telephone. If the problem is a desperate emergency, then ask for help straight away. In most cases, though, if the doctor or nurse is busy when you call and you simply want advice, ask if they will phone you back. Occasionally parents complain that the doctor isn't available to take the call right away. But think about it. Next time you are yourself in with the doctor discussing a worry or problem, would you really want the doctor to take phone calls right through your consultation? It makes far more sense for the doctor to speak to you between patients.

When to call the doctor

You should always consult the doctor if:

- You are worried and don't know what is wrong
- A child who has been vomiting looks drowsy or confused
- A child is pale, sweaty, and frightened
- A child has a stiff neck which hurts to move
- A baby under one year is listless or quiet, hot or floppy, or has an unusual cry
- A child has difficulty breathing, or a persistent cough
- A child has a convulsion
- A child develops a limp

CALLING THE DOCTOR

When you telephone your surgery or health centre you need to be ready with some clear information. The doctor and practice team receive a large number of calls throughout the day, and they need to be able to put them into some order of priority. If you simply say something like, 'I would like the doctor to visit,' then he or she really can have no idea as to whether this is an urgent life-threatening emergency, or a more minor difficulty. The reception staff should not quiz you for medical details, but it will help the medical team tremendously if you give:

- Your name and address
- Your phone number
- Your child's name
- What appears to be wrong with your child
- How urgent you believe the problem is
- Whether you need a home visit or just telephone advice
- Whether you need to speak to the doctor *now*, or whether it can wait till later

Obviously, every consultation – whether in person or by phone – is different. When you see or speak to the doctor for advice, it is important to realise that you may not be offered a prescription on every occasion. After all, the commonest childhood health problems are infections. The vast majority of childhood infections are caused by viruses, and virus infections are not helped in any way by antibiotics, or indeed by any other drug other than paracetamol, so please don't be surprised or disappointed if your doctor recommends simple measures such as paracetamol or fluids for your child's illness. Many parents feel upset if this happens, but I really must stress that this does *not* mean that your problem has not been taken seriously, or that the doctor does not believe how worried you are. It simply means that in the doctor's judgement antibiotics, or similar drugs, will do nothing to help speed your child's recovery.

Incidentally, on behalf of the nation's doctors, may I ask

you to ensure that the person making the telephone call actually knows the details of what is wrong. An all-too-frequent occurrence is for the mother to care for the child all day, and for the father to call the doctor when he gets in from work. If the father doesn't know anything other than the fact that the child is unwell, and has to check with his partner for the answer to every question that the doctor asks, then this is a perfect recipe for a long, drawn-out, and not particularly efficient phone call.

Outside routine surgery hours, more and more doctors now work in out-of-hours 'doctors' co-ops'. These are groups of trained G.P.s who share their on-call, and who are often based at an out-of-hours medical centre. Doctors are no longer obliged by their contract to visit other than for medical reasons (if the child has an infectious disease, for example), and you may well be asked to transport your child to see the doctor. There are many advantages in this system. The doctor you will see will be fresh, and working in a fully staffed and equipped medical centre. Whilst patients and parents often yearn for access to their 'own' doctor, available on-call for them twenty-four hours a day, every day, the ever-increasing volume of out-of-hours work means that this is frequently no longer possible, nor safe. In the same way as you would not like to fly in a plane with an exhausted sleep-deprived pilot, neither should you want to see a doctor in surgery who has been up dealing with minor medical problems and emergencies half the previous night.

However, one side effect of the increasing use of 'co-ops' is that the doctor you see will not have access to your child's medical records. So, when you speak to the doctor on the phone or attend the out-of-hours centre, do make sure the doctor knows about any allergies or significant past medical problems.

'If in doubt, ask' would seem to be the ideal summary. Remember that *you* are the expert on your child. Wise doctors listen to parents, and will share with you the reasons why they choose a particular course of action for your child. Going to the doctor should be a learning experience for parents. No one expects first-time parents to be instant experts on child health, but talking to your doctor, health visitor, and practice nurse – not to mention other parents – will give you a wealth of experience that will help you in the future.

HELPING THE DOCTOR EXAMINE YOUR CHILD

Most general practitioners become extremely skilled at examining children, though there are, sadly, a few exceptions. A large proportion of a G.P.'s workload is taken up with dealing with children, and the more skilful and kind the doctor is, the easier he will find the task. One famous paediatrician used to write 'If the child cries, it is my fault.' Whilst there is a great deal of truth in this statement, it is also true that careful and thoughtful preparation by the parent can make a remarkable difference.

Take two children who were brought to see me only last week. The first was a four-year-old lad whose mother was concerned that he might have an undescended left testicle. However, she had not told him what the consultation was about, so he arrived very reluctantly in my room, terrified about what was going on, uncertain about what I was going to do, and very reluctant indeed to lower his pants. The consultation was not easy. Nor was it particularly successful.

By contrast, the second child had been fully prepared by his mother. She was concerned that his foreskin was too tight. She had told him why he was being brought to see me. She had explained what I would do. And she also told me what their family name for his penis was (his 'winkle', as you ask) so that I was able to talk to him about what I needed to do, in terms that he could understand. Whilst he was understandably none too delighted to have someone studiously examining his winkle, he was remarkably co-operative, and I was able to compliment him on how good I thought he had been when I had finished.

So – preparation of your child can and does make a great deal of difference if your child is old enough. Be as honest as you can. After all, if you know your child is going to need an injection, then to say that you are just going to talk to the doctor is an outright lie, and will leave the child deeply mistrustful and frightened the next time a trip to the doctor is mentioned, however innocent this might be.

If you are nervous of seeing the doctor, then please do try to avoid teaching your child to be nervous in the same way. What do I mean by teach? Well, quite often I hear parents outside my consulting room saying things like, 'And if you're good, I'll buy you some sweeties afterwards.' What better way is there of teaching a child to expect something to be unpleasant? Would you ever offer sweeties as a behavioural bribe to a child who was off to the zoo, or to McDonald's? Of course you wouldn't. So, the child soon realises that the doctor's must be something unpleasant, or else his or her parents would not be offering such inducements.

Try instead to treat a trip to the doctor's as just one of those things. Your child will be far more relaxed, which will probably make things much easier for the doctor, which will make the next time even easier, and so the whole thing becomes the opposite of a vicious circle.

There are a number of specific tips that I can also give you as to how to make the consultation go well. These are based on over twenty years of having children as patients.

Clothing

Think about this in advance. If you know that the doctor is going to have to examine your little girl's abdomen, then bringing her to the doctor wearing a one-piece 'body' that is a real fiddle to undo, is less than ideal. Baby-gros are marvellous items of clothing for small babies, but are not always the ideal choice for a trip to the doctor.

Nappies

If your child is still in nappies, then do take a spare with you to the surgery. The simple truth is that, as sure as eggs is eggs, your baby will fill his or her nappy while you are in the waiting room. A spare nappy does make life much easier.

Ear examining

Doctors obviously get very used to examining children's ears, as ear infections are one of the most frequent causes of a trip to the doctor's. However it is not always terribly easy!

With babies and young children, the key to success is how the child is held. Sit your baby on your knee, so that he is facing to one side. Then use one hand to hold his head firmly against your chest, with your other arm wrapped gently around his upper body and arms, holding him against you. To examine the other ear, face him the other way and swap the arms holding his head and body. Do this, and your child will feel secure and confident, which means he can't wriggle, and this means that the procedure should be completely painless.

Throat examination

Children tend to hate it when doctors use tongue depressors – the wooden 'lollipop sticks' that some doctors use to hold the tongue down so that they can get a good view of the tonsils. Feeling the stick in the back of the throat can make some children gag, and be reluctant to be examined again.

In my experience, for the great majority of children there is no need for the doctor to use a tongue depressor *if* the child is able to open his or her mouth wide enough. With practice, most children can manage this. So – if your child is old enough – why not practise this before you go to the doctor. Often, saying that the doctor needs to be able to see the teeth right at the back is a good way of getting through to your child how much he or she needs to 'open wide'.

I'm not pretending that trips to the doctors are necessarily going to be easy or fun, but with preparation and kindness from both sides, most children don't need to feel apprehensive. Even playing with a toy doctor kit before you go can greatly help to prepare your child for what he or she should expect. Investing a little time in advance can pay great dividends.

Section Three

Childhood Symptoms

The child with a fever

Symptoms

Having a fever simply means having a temperature above normal. A normal temperature is defined as being 37°C or 98.4°F. However, children do vary slightly and many do seem to have a temperature that is always slightly less than this typical normal value. Sometimes you will simply know that your child has a temperature because he or she is so hot, but at other times you may need to use a thermometer.

Apart from having a raised temperature, other symptoms of fever may include shivering or feeling cold, or sweating and feeling hot.

There are several types of thermometer that you can use to record your child's temperature. The simplest by far are the forehead temperature-sensitive strips. These have the advantage of tremendous simplicity and safety. They are easy to read, and are the easiest to use with a wriggling uncooperative child. If this all makes them sound the ideal form of thermometer, they do – sadly – have the not-inconsiderable disadvantage of being notoriously unreliable. At best they give a guide to your child's possible temperature.

Traditional mercury-filled thermometers are accurate, but difficult to read. They consist of a glass tube containing a fine column of mercury. As the temperature goes up, the mercury expands along the column, and the actual temperature can be read off the calibrations next to the mercury. However, most people have to squint at them for quite a while before they can work out just where the top of the mercury column is. It is also essential to shake the mercury column down between readings. If you don't do this, the reading will be entirely meaningless. It is also essential to leave the thermometer in place until the reading is no longer changing. A few seconds will be useless. Ideally you should wait for two to three minutes, though this can seem like a lifetime with a restless child.

Some of the easiest and most accurate forms of thermometer are the newer electronic digital thermometers, which are battery powered and so do carry the slight risk of having flat batteries – though I have used one regularly for the past twelve months without the slightest sign of loss of power. They are extremely accurate, and reach the correct temperature much more quickly than mercury thermometers.

Traditionally medical advice books have suggested that the best way of taking the temperature is by inserting the thermometer in the child's rectum. If you really do need to record the temperature to the nearest fraction of a degree, then this is required, but for a simple guide as to whether your child has a temperature or not, I always recommend using the armpit if the child is too young to be co-operative, and the mouth, under the tongue, if the child is old enough. I usually use the armpit in children under five, and the mouth in older children, but this is not a strict rule. A useful tip is not to take the oral temperature shortly after a hot drink. You may be horrified by the result, which will be meaningless!

If you have been advised by your doctor to take the rectal temperature, then do check with your pharmacist that your thermometer is safe for this purpose, and always use lubricating jelly, such as Vaseline or KY Jelly, before you attempt to insert it.

Causes

Fever is a symptom, not an illness. It is almost always the result of an infection with either viruses or bacteria. A raised temperature is part of the body's normal response to such infection and is almost certainly part of the way in which the body attempts to fight off the offending organisms. Indeed, there are those who argue that by treating a fever we are prolonging the infection. Whilst this might theoretically be true, it is also not a particularly kind argument. Children with a high fever feel ill, and may even have a fit – known as a febrile convulsion. In general, therefore, it is both kind and sensible for parents and carers to attempt to lower the child's temperature back to normal – though do remember that all you are doing is making the child feel better, you aren't actually getting rid of the infection itself. This will take time, the body's natural defences, and, if necessary, other treatments.

Whilst infections are by far the major cause of raised temperatures, occasionally a consistently slightly raised temperature can be a sign of some other inflammatory problem such as arthritis, or bowel inflammation.

When to consult a doctor

As a doctor I am usually less interested in precisely how high a child's temperature is, than how ill he or she is. Indeed, on the majority of occasions I never take the temperature at all because I know it won't change my course of action. If the child is well and happy, I won't want to treat him or her, and if the child is unwell then I will want to find out why. However taking the temperature can sometimes be a useful guide in unravelling an otherwise confusing clinical picture. For instance, the child with tummy ache who has a raised temperature is slightly more likely to have appendicitis than the child whose temperature is normal – though this is only one of a number of clues.

So, if your child seems very sick, consult a doctor whatever the temperature. If your child has a temperature higher than 39.5°C or 102.5°F then you really would be wise to seek medical advice, though significantly high temperatures are actually very common at the start of many childhood illnesses. You should seek medical help immediately if a baby has a temperature of over 104°F (40°C).

How you can help

The single most important thing that you can do with a hot child is cool him or her down. That may sound ridiculously trite, but countless parents ignore it. Like all doctors I regularly see children with sky-high temperatures who are effectively being cooked by their parents. I visit them at home to find them fully dressed, wrapped in a thick blanket, and often sitting in front of a roaring fire. Nothing is more guaranteed to keep the temperature high.

Parents are often frightened that if they don't keep their child wrapped up, then he or she will develop a chill. I'm not quite sure what a chill actually is! Indeed I am absolutely certain that chills don't really exist, and that cooling can do no harm whatsoever.

Very many parents who bring their child to the doctor's surgery are often embarrassed that the child is so much better when they arrive. 'But he was really poorly half an hour ago,' they complain, 'and now look at him.' I am certain that the children feel better because the trip out to the surgery has cooled them down. I know that many parents are still very reluctant to take a child with a temperature out of the home to see the doctor, but in fact the journey can do no harm at all.

If your child is hot, cool him or her down. Firstly, remove most of the child's clothes – possibly just leaving on a thin vest or nightie. If necessary a cooling fan can be helpful, though this should not be aimed directly at the child. Cool sponging or even giving a cool bath – cool, not cold – can also help tremendously and be very soothing. As the water evaporates from your child's hot skin, it will cool the skin very effectively. Don't forget the importance of cool drinks which can also make a significant difference.

Finally, don't forget the importance of rest. Everyone recovers quicker from infections if they rest. As adults we often battle on when we shouldn't. If we can't treat ourselves properly, then we can at least give our children the benefit of rest!

Treatment

As far as medication is concerned, by far the most important and valuable is paracetamol. Aspirin is no longer considered safe in children aged under twelve, and should never be given. Paracetamol can come under a number of trade names such as Calpol, Disprol, or Panadol – and also comes in numerous other forms. To be honest, every brand of paracetamol is as effective as any other brand. Choose the cheapest formulation that has a flavour which your child will take. Despite all the hype, the expensive brand names are no more effective than the cheaper alternatives, and carry no other important ingredients other than flavourings. The chief alternative to paracetamol is ibuprofen, with alternative brand names including Junifen, Brufen, and Nurofen.

As well as lowering the temperature back towards normal,

these drugs also act as pain killers, which are tremendously useful in conditions such as a sore throat. Ibuprofen is also an anti-inflammatory drug. They are available mainly as syrups, and I would always recommend that you choose the sugar-free form. Paracetamol is remarkably free from side effects, provided the specified dose is not exceeded, and ibuprofen is valuable and safe for most children, though is not advised in children with asthma as it can sometimes worsen wheezing.

Prevention

Sadly, there is not much you can do to prevent your child from getting a fever – but you can prevent the temperature rising too quickly too fast by using the tips I have given above.

The child who is in pain

For any parent, seeing their child in pain is always a distressing experience. None of us likes to see our child suffer, and we all feel desperate to help. I will never forget one of the most distressing few hours in my life as a parent. As a family we were on holiday in Sardinia, and on the very last day – a few hours before we were due to catch the plane – my daughter began to complain of abdominal pain.

I examined her abdomen and thought that it could, just could, be appendicitis. But I didn't know whether I was over-reacting or not. The average parent would probably have given a spoon of medicine and finished packing, but as a doctor I found myself at a total disadvantage. I knew if I involved another doctor that Katy would end up being admitted to a Sardinian hospital, and would have her appendix removed that evening. I knew that at least fifty per cent of girls who are admitted to hospital with appendicitis turned out to have an entirely normal appendix, so any such operation might be unnecessary. But at the same time I couldn't help but wonder what would happen if her appendix became gangrenous and perforated in the plane at 35,000 feet. How would I cope then? Watching her lying on her bed holding her stomach, I began to feel sick with apprehension and anxiety. My poor wife was reduced to having two incapable invalids on her hands!

As it happened, the pain did gradually subside before the plane touched down at Gatwick, and she still has her appendix to this day. But yet again, I found the experience of anxiety about my own child taught me more about parenthood and childcare, than any number of lectures at medical school.

Symptoms and causes

This chapter will only deal with the general principles involved in an understanding of pain. Specific pains will be dealt with in different chapters, and you can find where to look in the index. There are countless possible causes of pain, and some of the commonest are:

Infection: such as the pain of an ear infection or abscess
Trauma: such as the pain from a twisted ankle or broken finger
Inflammation: such as the pain of arthritis or of nappy rash

In addition, every pain has two main components – the physical and the psychological – and both of these are important. Think of something as simple as a twisted ankle. If you were to twist your ankle just before you were leaving on an exciting holiday trip abroad do you think it would hurt more or less than the same twist happening just before a trip to the dentist for root canal work? The psychological component of pain can be tremendously important. Fear, apprehension, and anxiety can greatly worsen a pain. Reassurance and calmness can relieve it. Every doctor knows of patients in apparently agonising pain whose pain is relieved almost totally by a calm reassuring manner and belief in the medication, the pain often disappearing before any active constituent of the drug could have begun to take effect.

In addition, some pains are purely psychological. I am sure that you have suffered from headaches that are purely caused by a very stressful day and anxiety. Children tend to get tummy aches that are their equivalent of an adult's headaches. Most parents become used to their child having 'Monday-morning tummy aches' before school, or similar symptoms. However, no recurrent pain should ever be blamed on psychological causes unless a doctor has had a chance to assess and examine the child. Recurrent tummy aches, for example, may be the sign of a persistent slight urine infection, and detecting and treating this is vitally important.

When to consult a doctor

The child who is in pain is one of the very commonest reasons for parents to visit a doctor. A doctor's first job when faced by someone in pain is to try to work out what the cause of the pain is. To do this, he or she will start by asking a large number of questions. Older children will be able to answer these, but for younger children the parent is the only one who can answer. The areas that will be covered include:

- Where is the pain?
- What type of pain is it – sharp, dull, aching, stabbing, etc.?
- Does it spread anywhere?
- Does anything make it worse? (Such as eating, breathing, coughing, moving.)
- Does anything make it better? (Such as changing position, having the bowels open, etc.)
- What other symptoms are there? (Cough, sore throat, vomiting, etc.)
- Is your child otherwise ill, or does he or she seem to be happy and well apart from the pain?

In addition, the doctor will be interested in knowing what

you as a parent think might be going on. Wise doctors realise that parents are the experts on their own children, but in addition, the doctor needs to know what you might be frightened of if he or she is to reassure you. For instance, a parent might be convinced that a particular set of symptoms means that the child has a heart problem, but not actually expressing this fear to the doctor. The doctor may rapidly come to the conclusion that there is some other cause. If the doctor doesn't know that the parents are worried about the heart, he or she may not mention it. And if the doctor doesn't mention it, the parent may think that the doctor hasn't even considered the matter and thus been able to rule it out. So, if your doctor says 'What do you think might be causing this?' please don't say 'I thought it was your job to tell me, doctor' – a phrase that drives doctors to distraction.

Taking the history – in other words, asking questions about the pain – is the most important part of trying to unravel the cause of a pain. Scientific research has shown that over eight out of ten diagnoses are made using information gained from the history alone. Physical examination contributes the great majority of the remaining diagnoses, and special tests such as X-rays are only needed in a very small minority of cases.

How you can help

Obviously, the most important way you can help is to find out what the cause of the pain is and deal with this specifically. In addition, some pains can be eased by applying a hot water bottle, or massaging the affected area gently. If you use a hot water bottle, make sure that it is covered, or is not so hot that there is a risk of burning the skin. If your child is old enough, he or she will be able to tell you what helps most.

Treatment

For all pains there can be a place for general pain-relieving medication. Paracetamol and ibuprofen are the two most important pain-relieving drugs used in children, and I give full details of these in the appendix to this book. You should never use aspirin in children under twelve.

The child who is crying

Symptoms

The simple fact is that all babies cry. Crying is normal. It is a tiny baby's only means of communication. Adults cry when they are upset, or occasionally if they feel very moved by something, but babies cry when they are hungry, thirsty, cold, hot, lonely, wet, or any one of a hundred different reasons. New parents in particular often assume that the tears mean that their child is in deep distress, as they know that they themselves would only cry if things were really bad. But it isn't necessarily the case.

Incidentally, the bulk of this chapter will only be dealing with crying babies. Older children who cry should be considered in the same way that you would consider a crying adult. Something is clearly going to be significantly wrong, and most children who are old enough to talk will be able to explain what their problem is. The older child who sits and cries for no very apparent reason, and who constantly feels lethargic and miserable, may possibly be suffering from a clinical form of depression and you should certainly seek medical advice.

However, there is also no doubt that some babies cry an awful lot more than others. They cry, and they cry, and they cry, and they cry, and just when you think that they can't have the energy left to cry any more, they start crying again. When my son was a baby, he was one of the most miserable creatures on earth until he reached the age of seven months. Survival sometimes felt as if it could be touch and go. Then, when he had found how to move around, the tears suddenly dried up and have rarely returned since. But my wife and I certainly know what the parents of persistent criers have to put up with.

Whole books have been written on the topic of persistently crying babies, and a short section in a book like this can only begin to scratch the surface. The simple fact is that some babies are just much more placid than others, and the amount that they cry varies as much as the amount adults talk.

Parents generally become very expert in noticing differences in their child's crying, even if to other people one crying baby sounds much like any other. Many mothers can distinguish between the cry that says 'I'm hungry' and the one that says 'I'm lonely'. Parents often take their baby to the doctor saying that 'I know that something is wrong by the way he's crying,' and the wise doctor will always take note of this.

The parents of a crying baby often feel guilty, believing that if their baby continues to cry then they must be doing something wrong. If you can't comfort your child then it does make the whole experience seem much worse. After all, it can be incredibly difficult to know what the tears are about, particularly because there is often no simple answer.

With newborn babies, parents feel particularly vulnerable. This feeling of guilt and incompetence is often compounded by repeated sleepless nights. The early weeks and months of parenthood can sometimes be the perfect recipe for misery, even in the most dedicated, loving, caring and competent of parents.

The time when most crying occurs is during the first twelve weeks of life. Studies have shown that at six weeks, a quarter of babies will be crying or miserable for more than three hours a day. Interestingly this finding applies across the world. It isn't just restricted to Western cultures and may indeed be what is normal for all of humanity.

The worst time of day is the between six p.m. and midnight, with nearly a half of crying time being in this time slot. Recent research into crying has shown that at three months of age, two hours of crying a day is quite typical, and more than three hours each day is actually quite common. The good news is that this does generally get much better by the time the child reaches one year of age, and that many will be much better well before this.

Causes of persistent crying

If all babies cry, it is perfectly possible that the worst criers are just at one end of the normal spectrum. After all, some babies are bigger, or have larger noses, or more hair, or whatever. For every human attribute, someone will have it to extremes, and crying behaviour may be just one example of this. In other words, it is possible that some persistent criers are not necessarily crying about anything at all, they may just be crying because that is what they do. Whilst this can be reassuring, it is also important to try to find out why your child is crying if you possibly can, but do realise that you may not come up with an answer.

Many people have thought that crying babies occur more with anxious, tense, less competent mothers. However, the good news is that there is absolutely no evidence for this whatsoever. Mothers who are faced with persistently crying babies may understandably become more tense and anxious, but this is as a result of having the crying child. It isn't the cause of the tears.

However, possible causes of tearfulness include any or all of the following: hunger, thirst, boredom, nappy rash, earache, teething, tummy ache, wet nappy, pain, over-tiredness, feeding problems (such as difficulty in latching onto the breast), feeling too hot or too cold, colic, and absolutely nothing at all! As I have already mentioned, some parents become skilled at distinguishing one cry from another, and can tell what the likely cause is from the pitch of the cry, although some children don't seem to alter pitch much at all, so it might be impossible to tell.

When to consult a doctor

If your baby seems unwell, and has a cry that sounds different from his or her normal cry, then you should consult a doctor without delay. Sudden onset crying in babies who don't usually cry also needs to be sorted out, unless the cause is immediately obvious to you.

Babies who cry all the time can be extremely worrying, and I believe that it is an important part of a doctor's job either to find the cause and treat it, or ensure that there is nothing wrong and offer reassurance and guidance. So, if in doubt, do consult your doctor – but don't feel guilty, or that this has been a waste of time, if it turns out that there is no serious cause. After all, if you leave the consulting room less worried than when you went in, then this cannot possibly be a waste of anyone's time.

Health visitors can also be a very real source of advice and guidance with crying children. They usually have a wealth of experience in advising parents, and can share this with you.

How you can help

The single most important aspect of dealing with a crying baby is to attend to the cause, if you can find one. If you can't pinpoint what is going on, then there are many tips that parents have learnt over the years that may help you.

Picking your child up and carrying him or her around can help a very great deal. Constant carrying of babies is actually very normal in many other cultures. An important Canadian study showed that babies carried for at least three hours a day cried less than the control group. Carrying your child in a papoose can be a simple way of achieving this, and still leaves you able to get on with housework or other activities.

Whilst I fully appreciate that this is not always practical, it can be very successful and there is certainly no evidence that it does any harm. As in so much else in parenthood, the most important message is that you should do what you believe in, and don't be bullied into raising your child in a way that feels wrong for you.

Most parents make the discovery that movement seems to calm crying babies. This may involve walking up and down pushing the pram, or you may need to drive the child round and round in the car. When my daughter was a baby, we frequently couldn't calm her at night and I spent many a happy hour in the middle of the night, driving her around the deserted streets – deserted that is except for other parents driving their babies around!

If, despite all your best efforts, the crying goes on and on and you feel yourself getting more and more desperate, then do ask a friend, relative, or someone else to help if this is at all possible. The combination of frustration, worry, and exhaustion can be a time bomb, and someone else may be able to give you the brief breather that you so desperately need. The excellent self-help group, Serene (formerly Cry-Sis), has a team of volunteers who offer telephone support and who can be a great source of strength to desperate parents. Their contact details are in the appendix to this book.

If it is absolutely impossible for you to get anyone to help and you are on your own with your crying and screaming baby, and you are at the end of your tether, then my advice is simple.

Put your baby down somewhere safe. Now leave the room for ten minutes. Your baby won't come to any harm over this time. Try to cool down. Take a breath of fresh air. Have a cup of tea or coffee, or even a cigarette if you absolutely must. Try some slow controlled deep breathing. Then, when you feel you have calmed down, return to the baby.

And if you have a baby who cries a lot and on whom a huge proportion of your time is spent, soothing him or her to such an extent that your house becomes a tip then – so what? It's all a matter of priorities. The crying will end. You can catch up with everything else later.

Treatment

This obviously depends on the cause of the crying. If your baby is crying with earache, then the relevant treatment is to tackle the earache – and details will be found in the relevant section of this book.

For the child who is in pain, paracetamol and ibuprofen can be extremely effective pain killers, and details are given in the appendix.

Prevention

Because we don't fully understand why some babies cry more than others, it is difficult to offer particularly helpful advice on preventing crying in the new baby. Some paediatricians have suggested that babies rapidly learn that crying is the best way to get attention and to get their own way, and that if parents intervene early – changing nappies very early for example – then they might be able to prevent it. However this is still very debatable. There is, as I mentioned earlier, some evidence that carrying your child round, or giving him or her lots of attention, may help prevent some children from crying.

One area where there is definite scientific evidence that you can prevent one type of crying, is in preventing the problem of the child who wakes repeatedly during the night and cries until he or she is fed. Many parents feed their child to sleep. This is very natural. You keep feeding until your child dozes off in your arms, and then gently lay the child down and tiptoe away. The problem with this is that the child has learnt that the natural way to get to sleep is to have something in his mouth such as a nipple or teat. When the baby wakes, he will cry and cry until the nipple or teat is replaced, and he can drift off to sleep again. If, however, parents gently wake their baby at the end of a feed and then lay the child down in the cot, he will drift off without anything in his mouth, and so when he wakes – which will inevitably happen during the night – he will be able to drift off again without needing any help from his mother. Not only does this make sense in theory, it has been shown to work in practice. But it can only help your next child – not the one who is crying now!

The child with a cough

Every child coughs at times. When considering the coughing child, we really need to look separately at two quite different problems – known in medical jargon as the acute and the chronic cough.

Most non-medical people use the word chronic to mean 'really bad' – as in having a 'chronic backache today'. In fact it actually means that a problem is long-term. Chronic bronchitis is bronchitis that has been going on for a long time, whilst acute bronchitis is a short sharp problem.

A cough can actually be a good thing. It is nature's way of clearing the chest, or preventing infection or irritation from reaching the chest. If you inhale a pea by mistake whilst eating a meal, the resulting cough shifts the pea and keeps it from becoming lodged in the airways. The cough that most of us get when going into a smoke-filled room has a similar purpose. I will consider all these various factors in the section on causes. However I am sure that you will see immediately that just giving a cough-suppressing linctus can actually be exactly the wrong thing to do, if the cough is actually being beneficial.

Symptoms

A cough will sometimes be fruity or loose, and will sometimes be dry – descriptions that I am sure will make immediate sense to everyone. The fruity, moist cough is most likely to be caused by some form of infection, whilst the dry cough may be caused by simple irritation (say from fumes or smoke, or possibly from the catarrh associated with a cold), or may possibly be triggered by asthma. Parents are often surprised if doctors diagnose asthma in children who just have a cough, with no wheezing.

Causes

Every cell in the body requires a regular and plentiful supply of oxygen. The function of the lungs is to allow oxygen to diffuse across the thin membranes in the smallest air passages into the bloodstream. At the same time they also allow carbon dioxide to be cleared out of the blood. Problems can occur with almost any part of this system.

Without a doubt, the simplest way to think of the anatomy of the airways in the lungs is as an upside-down tree. The trunk is the trachea, the main airway that runs down from the throat. The branches, or bronchi, then become smaller and smaller – becoming bronchioles, and alveoli – the equivalent of the tiniest twigs. At birth, the lungs have a mere twenty million alveoli, but by the age of eight years there will be about 300 million of these tiny tubes! The bronchi are lined with tissue that is very similar to the lining of the nose. Just as when you get a cold, the lining of the nose becomes swollen and congested, or alternatively the nose may run, the same happens with the lining of the air passages.

A cough is the body's way of trying to keep the lungs clear and clean. The cough reflex is protective. There are plenty of barriers that are designed to stop noxious substances getting into the lungs – the nasal hairs act as a filter, and the mucus in the lungs also has a protective effect. However, sometimes germs or irritants can get through, and the cough reflex comes into its own – trying to expel them again. With a bout of coughing the germs or chemical irritants, such as fumes, are coughed clear.

Coughing also helps to clear sputum from the lungs. Sputum, sometimes called phlegm, can either be mucus or pus. Mucus can be produced when the linings of the bronchi are inflamed when there is no infection present.

Anything that causes irritation to the airways can cause a cough. Sometimes this will be infection, as in bronchitis or bronchiolitis. Incidentally, any word ending in '–itis' means that inflammation or infection is the cause. Appendicitis is simply an inflammation of the appendix. Tonsillitis is infection of the tonsils. And so it is with bronchitis, bronchiolitis, or even tracheitis.

The word 'bronchitis' simply means infection of the bronchi, or 'chest infection'. Many patients and parents worry intensely if they are told that the diagnosis is 'bronchitis'. They are muddling this with the more significant problem of 'chronic bronchitis', a long-term repeating difficulty that particularly affects smokers.

DIFFERENT TYPES OF COUGH

Cough that is worse at night or after exertion

A cough that goes on and on, mainly at night, or on exercise, is quite likely to be caused by asthma. Indeed, there are many doctors who say that children with a persistent night cough have asthma till proved otherwise. This may puzzle you, particularly if your child never ever seems to wheeze and you have thought of asthma as being a problem characterised by wheezing. In fact, coughing is just as important a symptom in many children.

Indeed, you may be worried if your doctor diagnoses asthma and your child 'only' has a cough. The importance of the diagnosis is that it means the correct treatment will be given. Countless children are given one antibiotic after another for a cough, when all that may be required is a course of anti-asthma medication. There is a full description of the causes and treatments of asthma in the next chapter on 'The child who wheezes'.

The infant with rapid breathing and a dry cough

This may well be caused by bronchiolitis, a condition that occurs mainly in infants, and which doesn't occur in older children. It is caused by a virus known as R.S.V. (respiratory syncytial virus). The main symptoms of bronchiolitis are rapid breathing and dry cough. As in other virus infections, antibiotics are completely useless and don't help the cough. However, steam often does help relieve the child's symptoms. The doctor is quite likely to send your child into hospital if he or she is unwell. This is usually a very brief admission, but treatment can relieve the distressing symptoms very rapidly.

Whooping cough

This is a condition that is now rare – thanks to the highly effective immunisation programme, but it has very definitely not yet been eliminated. Parents often misunderstand what is meant by the term 'whooping'. It is not a whoop as the child coughs, but instead the whoop occurs with the intake of breath at the end of a spell of coughing. In other words, the typical symptom is 'cough, cough, cough, cough – whoop'.

It is a condition that is very serious in infants, which is why immunisation is so important. After a spell of coughing a lot of clear frothy mucus may come up in the nose and mouth. These spasms of coughing are painful and distressing to watch, and infants may well need hospitalisation. Prolonged coughing can lead to brain damage, or permanent damage to the lungs. Parents often worry about the dangers of immunisation. Please do not forget the very real dangers for a child in not being fully immunised. Incidentally, if your child is in contact with someone with whooping cough, he or she may be given an antibiotic called Erythromycin, which can help to prevent the condition taking hold.

Bronchitis and pneumonia

Whilst they might sound dramatic, bronchitis and pneumonia are simply terms for different types of chest infection. Pneumonia is actually remarkably common, particularly in children aged between four and ten years, but many doctors avoid using the word to patients as they know how frightening it can be.

The difference between these two conditions is fairly straightforward. Bronchitis means that there is infection of the air passages, whilst in pneumonia the actual tissue of the lung becomes infected as well. Sometimes these can really only be distinguished by a chest X-ray, but they both generally respond well and rapidly to antibiotics. The child with pneumonia is likely to be unwell, often with a fever, and may sometimes grunt as he or she breathes.

A cough which is associated with fever may well be a sign of bronchitis or pneumonia, particularly if it has lasted more than a few days – so do seek medical help.

Croup

Croup is a type of cough caused by infection of the throat and upper airways. Typically it starts remarkably suddenly, coming on completely out of the blue. The noise of croup can be terrifying. It sounds like a cross between a seal barking and a child choking (although the child is not actually choking at all).

Characteristically croup comes on in the middle of the night, and sometimes – though not always – follows a cold. Breathing in this condition is usually noisy. The child gets frightened and breathes even more quickly. A classic vicious circle then develops and the problem gets worse and worse.

A similar thing happens as a result of a raised temperature. The child often has fever. The higher the fever, the more rapid the breathing, and the worse the symptoms. It can all be very frightening – for child and parent alike.

Approximately one in every ten children with croup is admitted to hospital, and of these one in twenty needs active medical intervention to keep the airways clear or to treat respiratory failure – an extremely serious condition.

The main first aid treatment for croup is steam – described clearly in the 'How you can help' section – but your child may need urgent medical attention too. The great majority of cases of croup get better without specific treatment, but if the symptoms are severe enough doctors are increasingly giving treatment using a nebuliser – a device (usually electrical) that creates a fine mist of moisture containing the relevant drug. The two drugs that are most used in this condition are adrenaline and budesonide (a form of steroid). Nebulised adrenaline should only ever be given in hospital, and under very close supervision. However the inhaled steroid may well be given by your family doctor either before, or instead of, admission to hospital in less severe cases.

The child with a persistent cough

If a cough goes on for longer than a month, it could be

described as being 'chronic'. By far the commonest cause of a chronic childhood cough is asthma. This is discussed fully in the section on 'The child who wheezes'. Most doctors are likely to X-ray any child who has had a cough for several weeks. The main purpose of this is to exclude the collapse of part of a lung, which can follow the child inhaling a foreign body, such as a peanut or bead.

Other possible causes of chronic cough include a sinus infection, which can happen in children without them getting the headache that is so typical of adults with sinusitis. Increasingly common is a chest infection called mycoplasma, otherwise called atypical (unusual) pneumonia. Once it has been diagnosed, it is relatively straightforward to cure with the correct antibiotic.

Some children with a chronic cough may have an acute condition known as bronchiectasis. This typically follows an untreated chest infection, or a chest infection associated with a condition such as measles. The walls of the alveoli are damaged, and lose their natural elasticity, resulting in a chronic infection and a very fruity cough when an infection is present.

Finally, a relatively rare, but extremely important, genetic condition which can present as a persistent cough is cystic fibrosis. Typically this is associated with other medical problems, such as loose stools and failure to gain weight. Cystic fibrosis affects about one child in every 2,000 and tends to run in families. Unfortunately, It is beyond the scope of this book to go into the problem in detail. The charitably funded support group for this condition is the C.F.Trust, which can provide excellent information.

When to consult a doctor

Small babies

A cough in the first few weeks can cause more problems than a cough later in life. Not only do babies have tiny air passages, but their cough is also relatively weak, and is not much use at expelling germs or other irritants from the airways.

With an infant you should seek medical advice if:

- The cough lasts more than a couple of days
- The cough is associated with a raised temperature
- Your baby is off his or her food
- You are concerned that your baby seems to be unwell in any other way

Older children

In older children, you should see a doctor if:

- Your child is unwell with the cough
- Your child coughs mainly at night, or on exercising
- The cough started after an episode of choking (he or she may have inhaled a foreign body – such as a peanut, or bead, or sweet)
- A cough that followed a cold goes on for more than a couple of weeks

Croup

Severe croup can be a medical emergency. If you have followed the advice I have given above, and the croup is not settling, then you need medical help urgently. The clues you should look for are:

- If you simply cannot make your child comfortable, and particularly if he or she seems agitated

- If your child is too breathless to be able to speak
- If your child cannot swallow, and seems to be dribbling saliva
- If he or she looks ill – either pale, or grey, or even blue
- If the space between the ribs is drawn in with each breath

In these circumstances, contact a doctor immediately. If there is going to be a significant delay in the doctor either speaking to you or getting back to you, it is entirely justified to go immediately to hospital – provided your local hospital is equipped to deal with emergencies. Not all hospitals are, and it is a dreadful waste of precious time to go to the wrong unit.

Sputum Samples

In treating adults and older children, the doctor may ask you to try to obtain a sample of sputum, for examination at the laboratory to try and find out what particular bacteria may be causing any chest infection. However, children under six are almost never able to cough the sputum up and out, and they nearly always swallow it, so most experienced G.P.s don't ask for a specimen unless it really is essential.

How you can help

How you can best help a coughing child obviously depends on the cause of the cough, and will also be influenced by the age of the child in question.

With small children and toddlers, persistent coughing may be soothed by a steamy atmosphere. This can also be very helpful indeed in croup. Steam can be used by taking the child into a shower room or bathroom, and leaving the hot water running. This is the ideal method, but if this isn't practical, leaving an electric kettle boiling in the room can have the desired effect. If you have a kettle with an automatic cut-off, you can usually keep it boiling by leaving the top off. But two words of warning! Don't do this close to wallpaper that might peel in the steam. And make sure there is enough water in the kettle to prevent the element burning out.

Croup needs more than just steam. Children with croup do get extremely frightened, and calm reassurance can make the world of difference. However, if croup does not settle very rapidly, seek medical help right away, or take your child to the nearest casualty unit.

For non-croupy coughs in the toddler and older child, warm drinks can be very soothing. My favourite is hot blackcurrant juice, but everyone has their own personal choices.

Treatment

The treatment of a coughing child also depends on the cause. If your doctor diagnoses a chest infection, then antibiotics may well be prescribed. These are described in considerable detail in the appendix.

If the underlying cause is asthma, then your doctor is likely to prescribe inhaled medication. This too has a section in the appendix.

However, if the cough is just a simple tickle with no underlying cause, there may be a case for using a mild cough medicine. The best, and very definitely the cheapest, is simply described as 'simple linctus B.P.'. This causes very few side effects and can soothe an irritating tickle. If you require a linctus that is more powerful at suppressing a cough, then pholcodine linctus is acceptable. Talk to your doctor or pharmacist about the safe dose for your child's age.

One very important rule when dealing with a child with a cough is not to use any sedation to help the child sleep. There is a risk that this could interfere with breathing.

Prevention

Apart from avoiding smoking, there are a number of things that you can do to prevent your child repeatedly developing coughs. There is some evidence that breast-fed babies are less likely to develop asthma early in life. Obviously it may be too late this time, but this can be worth bearing in mind if you plan to have more children in the future.

Immunisation against pertussis is essential for almost every child. If you have any doubts about this, discuss it fully with your family doctor. There really are tremendous risks for the child who develops whooping cough, but despite this there are parents who seem to believe that all the risks are associated with the vaccine, rather than the condition. This simply is not the case.

A good diet, in particular taking plenty of fruit and vegetables, has also been shown to help, but by far and away the most important factor in preventing your child from having a cough is to make your house a no-smoking zone.

There is a very clear link between adults who smoke and children who develop chest infections. If you must smoke, smoke outside. Avoid smoking in the car if your child is with you. Smoke irritates the lungs, and a child who has some other form of chest infection or irritation cannot possibly be helped by inhaling tobacco smoke from other people in the house.

COMMON MYTHS ABOUT COUGHS AND CHEST INFECTIONS

- Contrary to common belief, bronchitis is no more serious than 'a cold on the chest'
- You cannot catch pneumonia from cold weather, being caught in the rain, or getting 'a chill'
- There is no such thing as 'double pneumonia'. It is a corruption of the term 'pleural pneumonia' which doesn't mean more than one pneumonia, but refers instead to the pleura – the covering of the lungs
- Treating a cold with antibiotics at the start will not stop the patient getting a subsequent chest infection

The child who wheezes

Symptoms

I am certain you will recognise a wheeze when you hear it. It is a high-pitched noise made by the lungs as the child breathes out. A noise made when the child breathes in is not true wheezing, and neither is the noise that children often make when they have a cold, but which disappears on coughing.

To understand the causes of wheezing you need to understand the basic anatomy of the lungs. As I explained in 'The child with a cough', you should think of the airways in the lungs as an upside-down tree. The trunk is the trachea, the main airway that runs down from the throat. The branches, or bronchi, then become smaller and smaller – becoming bronchioles, and alveoli – the equivalent of the tiniest twigs. The prime function of the lungs is to allow oxygen to diffuse across the thin membranes in the smallest air passages into the bloodstream. At the same time they also allow carbon dioxide to be cleared out of the blood.

Wheezing occurs because something obstructs the free flow of air. Imagine that you are blowing air through a short length of hosepipe. You will normally not be able to hear any significant sound as the air flows to and fro. However, if you pinch one end of the pipe to narrow it, you will hear the air as it passes through the obstruction. In the same way, anything that significantly obstructs air flow can cause wheezing.

Causes

The main causes of wheezing are bronchiolitis and asthma. Bronchiolitis typically happens up to the age of six months, whilst asthma becomes increasingly common after six months.

Bronchiolitis

Bronchiolitis (inflammation of the bronchioles) is a virus infection affecting babies, caused by the respiratory syncytial virus – the same virus that causes croup in older children. Commonest in the first six months of life, it can affect children up to eighteen months old. Typically the symptoms start with a cold, with a runny nose and possibly a slight fever. However, fairly rapidly the baby becomes wheezy, and this is frequently worse at night. Whilst it is usually a fairly mild condition, it can be severe and if you are concerned that your baby is struggling to breathe then don't hesitate – seek medical help urgently. Signs that your baby may be struggling to breathe include rapid breathing, going blue, in-drawing of the space between the ribs and below the lowest ribs, appearing distressed, and tightness of the muscles around the shoulders and neck.

Severe bronchiolitis is likely to need hospital admission, where the baby will be treated with oxygen and humidification, and possibly antibiotics if there is thought to be secondary infection. It is not unheard of, though quite unusual, for second bouts of bronchiolitis to occur.

Asthma

Throughout the whole of childhood by far the main cause of wheezing is asthma, and that is what the rest of this chapter will mainly concentrate on. However there are other possible causes, and it is true to say that 'all that wheezes is not asthma'. The other vitally important conditions that can be mistaken for asthma are epiglottitis, and an inhaled foreign body, and I deal with both of these separately at the end of this chapter. Indeed, if you think of the description of the lungs that I gave above, you will be aware that blockage of any level of the airway could be the trigger for wheezing. For instance, an inhaled peanut can lead to obstruction of one of the main bronchi.

The main problem that occurs in asthma is inflammation of the lining of the bronchi. The bronchi are lined with tissue known as mucous membrane that is very similar to the lining of the nose. When you get a cold, you are aware that the lining of the nose becomes swollen and congested, and the same thing can happen with the lining of the air passages. You will also be aware that many things other than colds can make the lining of your nose swell and run, including fumes, irritation, infection, sudden changes of temperature, and so on.

Exactly the same applies to the airways. Every one of us will wheeze if the conditions are right. I don't suffer from asthma, but put me in a room full of acid fumes and I will very definitely start wheezing. The only difference between me and someone with asthma is the level of irritation or stimulation that is required to cause the inflammation and to set the wheeze going. Our thresholds are different. For me it may be acid fumes. For an asthmatic it may be a few pollen grains. But the principle is identical. When there is asthma in a family, the threshold for wheezing in all other individuals in the family tends to be lower, and it doesn't take as much to set the wheeze going. Incidentally, asthma is very much more common in atopic families – families where there is a history of either eczema, hayfever, or asthma. However, just because your child has one of these conditions it does not make it inevitable that he or she will get the others.

The main irritants that will cause wheezing are:

- Infection
- Allergy
- Change of air temperature
- Emotion
- Exercise

For some children, one stimulus will be much more important than others. For instance, some children will wheeze if they run, whilst others may wheeze if exposed to pollen. I see a significant number of children who only really seem to wheeze when they get an infection, others whose wheezing is seasonal and linked to allergies, and so on. The pattern is unique to any individual. However, the effect is identical. The lining of the bronchi becomes swollen and inflamed and this obstruction to air flow tends to cause a wheeze.

When to consult a doctor

I believe that all children who wheeze should be assessed by a doctor. If the wheeze is severe – with your child being significantly out of breath – then you should consult right away, but if it is simply a nuisance then make a routine appointment with your doctor. It may be that your child just wheezes after exercise, or has a wheeze or cough that is worse in the early morning. Both of these can be helped, so don't shy away from consulting a doctor because you would 'rather not know that it was asthma', as one mother recently said to me. A tremendous amount can be done for asthma these days, and a correct diagnosis means that the correct effective treatment can be given, rather than repeated courses of antibiotics or other medication.

How you can help

The most important thing that you can do is be aware of wheezing, and seeking help when appropriate. In the early stages, if you are in any doubt about your child's symptoms, why not keep a diary for a week or two? Record exactly when the wheeze seems to happen. Is it at any particular time of day or night? Is it affected by exercise or excitement? Information like this can make it much easier for your doctor to make a correct diagnosis.

If the doctor does diagnose asthma, then find out as much as you can about it. Ask questions. Ask your doctor or practice nurse if they have any information booklets or leaflets about the condition. Understanding asthma makes a tremendous difference to how well it can be controlled or treated. Many general practices now run special asthma clinics, and should be able to discuss with you a wide range of treatment options – but don't be afraid to ask about them.

Treatment

In the appendix I cover the different types of drugs that can be used in asthma in very considerable detail, and I won't repeat myself here.

However, I would stress a few points:

- There is no such thing as a 'cure' for asthma. The aim of treatment is to control it, so that the child lives an entirely normal and active life. The majority of young children with asthma tend to grow out of it.
- Asthma is not a reason for a child to be any less active than his or her peers. If top sportsmen like Ian Botham

can be asthmatic, then there is no reason for asthma to stop your child enjoying sport.

- If your doctor prescribes a 'preventer' drug – usually a brown inhaler – then do use this regularly. The aim is to prevent symptoms happening. If you stop it when your child is well, symptoms are likely to flare up again.
- Your doctor may advise you to keep a 'Peak Flow Diary'. By using a special meter, available free to children on prescription, it is possible to measure accurately how wheezy, or normal, your child's breathing is. Regular recordings can help decide the correct form and potency of any treatment.
- There is no evidence that treatment stunts a child's growth. There is plenty of evidence that the child with poorly controlled asthma grows less well than other children. Good control matters.

Prevention

There is one golden, and rather predictable, rule for reducing the severity and frequency of asthma attacks (other than using the correct medication regularly). Make your house a no-smoking zone.

In addition, there is good evidence that being breast-fed reduces the likelihood of a child developing asthma. It doesn't make it impossible, but it does help.

Epiglottitis

Epiglottitis is extremely rare, but extremely serious. The epiglottis is the flap of cartilage at the back of the throat. Incidentally, despite what many people think, it is not the 'dangly bit' that you can see hanging down at the back of the throat which is actually the uvula. The epiglottis normally closes the entrance to the trachea when you swallow, so preventing food or drink from being inhaled.

Epiglottitis is an infection – usually caused by a virus – which leads to severe and sudden swelling of the epiglottis and which therefore interferes seriously with breathing. The typical symptoms are:

- The child suddenly becomes unwell and feverish, with a severe croupy cough.
- He or she may be struggling for breath, with drawing in of the muscles between and under the ribs, and flaring of the nostrils.
- The child may be unable to swallow anything at all – including saliva, so dribbling is a common symptom.
- As the condition worsens, the child becomes more and more breathless, with rapid breathing and a rapid pulse. If you suspect this, then seek medical help NOW. This is a genuine emergency. Incidentally, do NOT try and look in your child's throat as gagging can greatly worsen the condition.

Treatment at hospital includes oxygen, steroids, and possibly the insertion of a tube to by-pass the obstruction. This condition is rare – I have seen one case in over twenty years – but it is obviously vitally important.

Choking (inhaled foreign body)

Small children have a great tendency to inhale tiny objects – from peanuts and sweets, to tiny Lego bricks and beads. If your child is having difficulty breathing or has stopped breathing and you think that he or she has done this, then follow this advice:

Choking in babies under one year

- Kneel on the floor, and hold your baby over your leg or your forearm, so that his or her head is lower than his chest.
- Using the heel of your hand, give three or four sharp blows on to your baby's back, between the shoulder blades.
- If the foreign body shifts, fine. If not, turn your baby over, place your first and second fingers on the centre of your baby's chest just below the line of the nipples, and give four quick chest thrusts.
- If you can see the foreign body has moved into your baby's mouth, slide a finger in and gently scoop it out.
- If none of these methods has worked, start artificial respiration. If someone is with you make sure they send for a 999 ambulance now. If you are alone, go through the cycle of artificial respiration twice and then urgently call yourself before you start again.
- For a baby this age, straighten your baby's neck, lift the jaw very slightly, and cover the baby's nose and mouth with your mouth. Then blow just hard enough to move your baby's chest up and down, and keep this going at a rate of about twenty breaths per minute. After each breath, briefly lift your mouth away from your baby's mouth, to let the air escape before you repeat the cycle.
- Keep doing this until either your baby starts breathing spontaneously, or an ambulance arrives.

Choking in children over one year

- Perform the Heimlich Manoeuvre. This is performed as follows:

  A If your child is *upright* (sitting or standing), stand

behind him and place your fist just between the tummy button and the bottom of the breastbone. Put your other hand over your fist, and *pull* sharply upwards and inwards *four times in rapid succession*. This is like **a very vigorous bear hug**. This frequently and dramatically shifts the foreign body.

B If your child is *lying down*, you need to recreate the same movement. Kneel next to the child, put *one hand on the upper abdomen* between the tummy button and breastbone. Put your other hand on top of this. Then **push sharply upwards and inwards** four times. Gently open the child's mouth, and if you see the foreign body, scoop it out. If you don't see it, don't go digging around as you could easily push it back in.

- If your child is still not breathing, begin artificial respiration. Tilt your child's head back slightly, and lift the jaw so that it is slightly lifted forwards. Squeeze the child's nose, so that air cannot pass through it. Then put your mouth over your child's, and blow in so as to make the chest rise. You may only have to breathe quite gently. Allow air to escape between each breath. Keep going at a rate of about fifteen breaths every minute.

Make sure that someone sends for an ambulance right away. If you are alone, try not to panic. Do the whole cycle of artificial respiration twice, then send for a 999 ambulance. Then return to your child until either breathing starts spontaneously, or an ambulance arrives.

With both infants and older children, if they inhale a foreign body but are managing to breathe, or are coughing or choking, then please don't bang the child on the back as sometimes this can make the foreign body go further down into the lungs. Try and calm your child. The coughing may well shift the object, but if not go straight to hospital. If the situation gets worse, follow the advice I gave above. If he or she seems to be better, still go for a check-up to make sure the object has moved completely. Occasionally the foreign body becomes like a plug in an airway, and can lead to a form of pneumonia setting up in the lung past the blockage. Indeed, sometimes a child can inhale a foreign body and the first sign is a persistent cough. This problem can occasionally only be diagnosed by X-ray.

The child with a cold

Colds are incredibly common, as you will be all too well aware. Indeed, the average adult will typically get about four colds a year. Children do even worse. As they haven't yet built up their full immunity to conditions like colds, they get even more of them. Indeed, the average child will have about seven colds per year, and even more than this if either the child him or herself, or a brother or sister changes school.

The official medical term for a cold is 'coryza', which is a typical rather absurd example of a condition being given a medical name which is longer, harder to remember, and no more clear than the good old-fashioned term. Colds may sometimes be associated with a cough, and the whole problem of coughing is dealt with separately in the section on 'The child with a cough'.

Symptoms

The main symptoms of a typical cold are:

- Blocked or runny nose
- Streaming eyes
- Mild sore throat

In small babies the airways in the nose are so small that they can easily become blocked. The resulting cacophony of snorting and snuffling can be quite alarming, and the child can seem very distressed. However this is not usually half as bad as it seems. Young babies only breathe through their mouth when they cry, with the blockage of the nose leading to the sniffling and snorting. But they aren't really as ill as you would be if it was you making all that noise. After all it would take a much greater level of congestion to block an adult nose with its relatively large air spaces, compared to a child's with its tiny tubes.

In addition, babies find it very difficult to feed if the nose is congested. After all, it is almost impossible to suck if your nose is blocked. Parents often worry that their baby may stop breathing during sleep because of the congestion. In fact, this isn't the case. If the nose is completely blocked, he or she will automatically wake up and cry, and crying is a very effective way of taking down a large gulp of air.

Older children have bigger noses, which are much less easily blocked, and they will also have learnt how to breathe through the mouth. For this reason, colds – whilst an irritating nuisance – never appear quite so dramatic in older children as they do in babies.

Causes

Colds are virus infections. There are about 200 different cold viruses, but unfortunately they keep changing and are different from year to year. They are split into two main groups, known as rhino-viruses and coronaviruses. ('Rhino–' in medicine refers to the nose. Plastic surgery on the nose is a rhinoplasty. A rhinoceros has a big nose.) Because the culprit in colds is a virus, antibiotics are completely useless in treatment. No viruses are killed by antibiotics, which are only effective against bacteria.

Because the cold viruses keep changing, none of us ever gets really good long-lasting immunity. We may become immune to this season's virus, but this won't protect us from a changed virus in a few months' time.

Despite what generations of grandmothers have said, you cannot possibly catch a cold from sitting in a draught, or from getting a chill – whatever a 'chill' is. The virus is transmitted either by inhaling droplets that contain the virus when someone with a cold has coughed or sneezed near you, or from rubbing the eyes or nose with fingers that have the virus on. It is certainly possible to pick up the cold virus in this way from handkerchiefs, or towels.

When to consult a doctor

As stated above, the great majority of colds will last between five and seven days, though babies can stay snuffly for up to another week. For simple colds there really is little point in seeing a doctor. After all, no doctor will be able to do anything more than you can. However there are occasions when you should seek medical help. These include:

Persistent fever

You should get your child checked over if he or she has a fever of over 102°F (39°C) for more than twenty-four hours, or a fever less than this for three days or more.

Earache

This may well be a sign of an ear infection, though if your child says his or her ear hurts 'a bit' and isn't particularly distressed, there is no need to contact a doctor unless it fails to clear up. Earache is not always a sign of an ear infection. Simple congestion of the Eustachian tube can lead to pain, by causing an imbalance of the pressure on each side of the ear drum. This is exactly the same as the earache that occurs when you travel by air.

Vomiting

If your child is vomiting or won't drink, this may be a sign that this is more than just a simple cold. There could be some sort of infection elsewhere – such as a chest infection.

If your child seems unusually ill

If your child seems to be more significantly ill, and you are genuinely worried, then seek medical help.

Difficulty breathing

Problems with breathing, other than the simple sniffles mentioned above, could very rarely be the sign of a problem like epiglottitis. In this, the epiglottis – which is a flap of tissue that normally prevents food or drink entering the windpipe – swells dramatically and can obstruct breathing. Seek help now! Similarly, if your child starts to wheeze, and is not known to have asthma which you feel comfortable in coping with, or if your child is breathing more rapidly than normal, then this is not just a simple cold. You should seek medical help.

Delayed symptoms

If your child develops a high fever, or becomes unwell some days after the cold starts, this could be the sign of a secondary infection which may need antibiotics. A doctor should check your child to make sure. However, it is entirely normal to have a tickly cough or a runny nose for anything up to a couple of weeks after the cold.

It is important to realise that doctors cannot treat colds. If your child develops an ear infection or even pneumonia some days after starting with a cold, do not blame yourself for not seeking medical help earlier. Even if you had gone to the doctor straight away, he or she would have been just as helpless at treating it as you are. Doctors should not give antibiotics for colds 'just in case', as this will mean tens of thousands of courses of antibiotics being given unnecessarily, and a very real risk of resistance to these useful drugs developing even more quickly than is happening anyway. One of the perils of parenthood is that parents inevitably feel guilty if their child develops something needing medical treatment after having symptoms for several days. Unfortunately, there is simply no way of avoiding this. I remember with my own children that I found it quite impossible to judge in advance when they were going to need medical treatment such as antibiotics. In the same way, it is futile and illogical to be cross with a doctor if he or she says on one day that your child does not need antibiotics and a few days later changes his or her mind. Mystic Meg may be able to read the future. The rest of us can't!

How you can help

There is no cure for the common cold. If I had the secret to this medical mystery, I would no longer be writing this book and buying lottery tickets, I would be sitting on a sunny beach working out how to spend my fortune. Quite simply, whatever you do about a cold, it will usually last between five and seven days. Indeed, you could say that, with treatment, colds will clear up in a week. Without, they take seven days.

What is important in a child is to make them as comfortable as possible by controlling the symptoms, and by encouraging your child to drink as much fluid as possible.

Food isn't terribly important. If your child isn't hungry, don't worry. But do encourage drinking.

Treatment

Nasal congestion can be helped by using nose drops – but these should never be used for more than five days. Prolonged use of almost all over-the-counter nose drops, (with the exception of steroid drops such as Beconase) can result in a rebound reaction, in that when the drops are stopped the congestion comes back worse than it was at the start.

Hundreds of different proprietary cold preparations are marketed. Neither my wife, nor I, nor any of my family have ever used a single one of them, and we have certainly had our fair share of colds. Most doctors that I know take the same attitude, and don't waste their money on products they don't believe in. Indeed, there really is precious little evidence that they are any better than paracetamol, and fluids. Most proprietary preparations contain anti-histamines and these can actually have more side effects than benefits.

Steam can certainly help to ease congestion. If your child really does have bad nasal congestion, a steamy atmosphere can help. You can either achieve this in a bathroom or shower, or alternatively in the kitchen with an electric kettle. (Automatic cut-off devices can usually be over-ridden by leaving the lid off.) For the older child sniffing a bowl of very hot water that contains menthol crystals, Vick, Karvol, or such-like, can be very comforting – but do be careful that the bowl cannot be tipped over. (Colds get better. Burns can leave scars.) I have never been terribly convinced that aromatic substances that you put on a baby's pillow or vest are genuinely effective, but they are at least safe – provided you follow the instructions carefully.

If your child has a cough that is keeping him, her, or even you awake, then look at the section on 'The child with a cough' for advice.

Prevention

Just as there is no guaranteed cure for any cold, neither is there any sure-fire recipe for a cold-free life. Certainly there are those who swear by vitamin C, and those who take cod-liver oil, vitamin supplements, every mineral under the sun, and so on. If any of them really worked, we would all know about it. What is worthwhile is making sure your child has an adequate diet – a topic that I deal with fully in *Food Fights*, a companion book to this title. The older child who never has fruit or vegetables, or even fruit drinks, is bound to be less resistant than the child whose diet is more balanced.

There is also plenty of evidence that children get more colds if they live in households where someone smokes. If you or your partner smoke, give up now! There is no better gift for a child than a smoke-free environment to grow up in.

And if someone in the house has a cold, don't forget how the virus is transmitted. Hygiene is important, although even the most scrupulously clean, tidy, and attentive parents will still have children who have colds. Colds are simply a fact of life.

The child with a sore throat

Symptoms

Sore throats are tremendously common. They can obviously happen at every age, but it is unlikely that you will be able to tell particularly easily that a small baby has a sore throat, for the simple reason that he or she cannot tell you. Babies with sore throats often simply seem unwell, or may have a temperature. They may be off their food, they may be reluctant to swallow, but the symptoms will hardly be specific.

In older children the diagnosis is much easier. They are likely to complain of soreness in the throat, and possibly of difficulty in swallowing. They may also have enlarged cervical glands – the lymph nodes in the front of the neck – and may also complain of tummy ache. This is caused by a condition called mesenteric adenitis. When you get a throat infection, the glands in the neck swell up to prevent the infection from spreading. In the same way, the glands in the abdomen may swell and become inflamed, causing pain which can sometimes be quite severe, and is quite frequently mistaken for appendicitis.

Causes

Sometimes a sore throat will be caused by tonsillitis, but on other occasions it is not. Parents often become very confused about this. So, what is the difference?

The simple fact is that most sore throats are mild, and your child won't seem particularly unwell. A sore throat may be part of an ordinary cold, and your doctor may describe it as an 'upper respiratory infection'. However, in tonsillitis, the sore throat is likely to be much more severe. The tonsils themselves will be swollen and red, and may be covered with white spots of pus. In addition, your child may have a high temperature, lose his or her appetite, and seem generally under the weather.

Sore throats and tonsillitis can both be caused either by bacteria or by a virus. Many doctors believe that the nastier a sore throat looks, the more likely it is to be a bacterial infection. However this is probably not the case. Indeed, the only way that a doctor can be really sure of the cause of a sore throat is by taking a throat swab, and sending it away to the hospital to get it analysed.

In truth, doctors are seldom terribly concerned about knowing whether the cause of a sore throat is bacterial or viral because an accurate diagnosis is actually of precious little help. If the doctor does take a throat swab the result could easily take three or four days to come back, by which time the condition is likely to be clearing anyway.

When to consult a doctor

When your child has a sore throat, you should go to the doctor if:

- The sore throat is not showing any sign of improvement after four days
- The child has a headache or is particularly unwell
- The child develops earache
- The child comes out in a rash
- You can't keep the child's temperature down
- You are in any way particularly worried about the child's condition

How you can help

If your child is feverish, you should cool him or her down by removing some clothes, and if necessary by bathing him or her in tepid water. Offer plenty of drinks, but don't worry if your child doesn't want to eat – a day or two without food will do no harm. Giving paracetamol will help to keep his or her temperature down, and will soothe the soreness. Indeed, it is quite likely that this is the only treatment that will be needed.

Treatment

For most cases of sore throat, the advice that I have given above should be all that is required. However, if the symptoms don't settle after four days or so, or if there are other symptoms such as those I have mentioned above, you may well consult your doctor. Parents often get confused that one doctor may always prescribe antibiotics, whilst others seem very reluctant to do this.

Approximately seven out of ten cases of tonsillitis are caused by viruses, for which there is no effective treatment other than pain killers. If the infection is caused by bacteria, on the other hand, then antibiotics may be helpful. But – as I said earlier – the doctor cannot tell with certainty which sore throats are viral and which are bacterial.

Medical opinion on how to treat young children varies widely. Some doctors give antibiotics routinely to your child on the grounds that they *might* help and probably won't do any harm. Other doctors are more concerned that over-use of antibiotics may result in bacteria becoming more resistant, which could lead to more severe infections for children in the future. Some doctors prefer not to prescribe antibiotics at all, because they feel that they are not necessary.

The usual approach is a compromise. The doctor may reserve antibiotics for throat infections that have lasted four or five days with no sign of improvement. Your doctor may take other factors into account, too. If your child has a part in the school play, or if you are going on holiday the next day, he might decide to prescribe antibiotics.

Prevention

Some children do seem to get an awful lot of sore throats. They are more common in three- to six-year-olds than in any other age group, and many under fives suffer from repeated infections. This is probably because they haven't had time to build up any real immunity to infection, and yet they are coming into contact with more and more people (and germs!) as they start playgroup and school.

The good news is that typically your child's frequent infections should tail off dramatically by about six. Incidentally, there is no evidence that sore throats are hereditary – some people are simply more susceptible to germs than others.

However, there is very little that you can do to prevent repeated sore throats, apart from making sure that your child has a balanced diet with plenty of fresh fruit and vegetables, and the right amount of sleep. This will help to boost his or her resistance to infection generally. If he or she is a faddy eater, you may wish to give vitamin supplements although there is no real medical evidence that this helps.

It certainly isn't necessary to keep your child away from other children, or to stop him or her playing out in cold weather. Sometimes, prevention can be more upsetting to your child than the condition that you are trying to avoid.

Tonsillectomy

Twenty or thirty years ago, it was very common for young children to have their tonsils out to prevent further infection. Nowadays, we know that the great majority of children grow out of repeated sore throats by the time they are around six, and that in most people the tonsils shrink away to next to nothing.

For this reason doctors today are much more selective about whether to recommend a tonsillectomy. There is little point in putting your child – and you – through the worry of surgery if it isn't really necessary, and no operation should be considered lightly. But, if your child has suffered four or five attacks of tonsillitis a year over the last eighteen months, your G.P. may decide that he or she would be better off without tonsils.

Normally, E.N.T. surgeons prefer to wait until a child is at least four years old before carrying out a tonsillectomy. This is because younger children will often refuse to swallow solid food after the operation, and it is important for them to get back to swallowing as soon as possible, as eating solid food helps to keep the wound clean and prevent infection. However, swallowing at this time will be painful, so at first your child will need to take paracetamol when he or she eats.

The child with earache

Earache has to be the bane of many young children's lives. Typically, it comes on during the night. Your child will probably start to sob, whilst unhappily clutching at an ear. There can be few more miserable sights and sounds. If you yourself can remember ever having earache, you will be well aware of what a distressing pain it can be. And yet, despite the abject misery that it causes, you may find the doctor you consult simply advises that you should give your child paracetamol and a cuddle. This can leave parents feeling cheated, and even angry. This chapter will attempt to unravel the whole problem of earache, explain why it occurs, and look at the different treatments that are available, as well as giving first-aid advice for those early morning tear-stained examples of the joys of parenthood and childhood.

Symptoms

In a child who is old enough to tell you what is wrong, the symptoms of earache are all too obvious. The ear hurts! What more is there to say? However, in younger children, the symptoms are much less clear cut. Earache is almost always caused by some form of ear infection, and the symptoms in those too young to explain are those of the infection.

In babies these symptoms can include crying, screaming, being generally and vaguely unwell, having a fever, and even loose motions or vomiting. Many parents get to recognise the cry of a child with earache. It is often more a high-pitched wailing, that sounds quite different to many other cries. I have lost count of the parents who have consulted me saying, 'It's his ears again' and who are entirely right, despite their child being far too young to give any other clue. In other children it can be far harder to tell what is going on, and a trip to the doctor is required for a clear diagnosis.

Causes

Earache can be caused by a number of different problems. These are:

Middle ear infection (otitis media) – the commonest
Outer ear infection (otitis externa)
Congestion of the Eustachian tube
Pain referred from the jaw joint (unusual in children)

Before explaining how these problems can occur, I need to explain the anatomy of the ear. Many parents have only a vague idea of what goes on inside the ear, but it is fundamental to understanding how problems occur, and how they are best helped.

The ear needs to be thought of as having three main parts – the outer, middle, and inner ear.

The outer, curly, part of the ear is rarely the source of any problems. The curious shell-like design is a very effective way of trapping sound and directing it into the ear canal. The ear canal (external auditory meatus) is simply a tube lined with thin and sensitive skin, and at the end of the canal is the ear drum.

The ear drum (tympanic membrane) is very thin, and looks like tissue paper stretched across the end of the ear canal. When sound waves hit the ear drum, it moves and the movements are transmitted to the inner part of the ear by tiny bones – the hammer, anvil, and stirrup. Just behind the ear drum is an air-filled middle ear cavity, and a tube –

known as the Eustachian tube – runs from this cavity down to the back of the throat.

The inner part of the ear contains the apparatus that converts the impulses from the ear drum into impulses that can be understood by the brain as sound, and it also contains the semi-circular canals, which control balance.

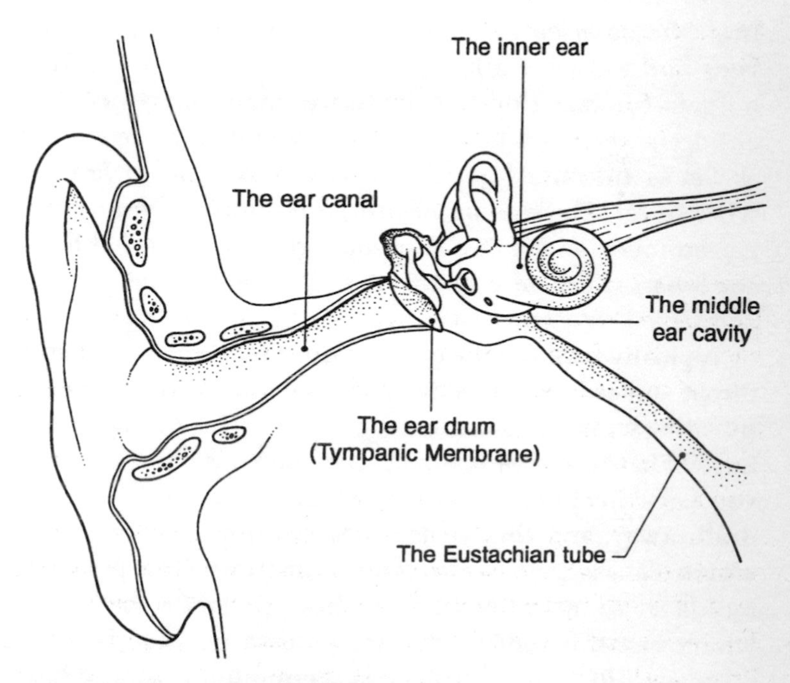

MIDDLE EAR INFECTIONS

Middle ear infection (or otitis media) is by far the commonest cause of severe earache in children. There is a one in three chance of any child having an episode of otitis media by the age of three years – but like all averages these figures disguise the fact that some children have very frequent infections.

These infections are commonest between six months and two to three years, become very much less common by the age of six, but can very occasionally cause problems up till the teenage years.

Middle ear infections occur because infection gets into the middle ear cavity through the Eustachian tube. It really is vital to realise this. The infection spreads from the throat to the middle ear up the Eustachian tube, and *not* inwards from the outer part of the ear. This explains why getting your child to wear a hat makes no difference to whether he gets ear infections. Countless parents insist on their children wearing a hat or muffler to protect the ears, but as far as infections go this simply makes no difference whatsoever. There is no need to feel guilty if your child has an infection the day after you forgot to insist that he or she wears a hat on a windy day. The two things are not connected.

Typically most middle ear infections follow a cold or sore throat. Indeed, ear infections are not themselves directly infectious. As the infection builds up, the lining of the Eustachian tube swells – just like your nose blocks when you have a cold. The pus in the middle ear cavity cannot drain away, and this leads to pressure on the ear drum which causes pain or earache. Sometimes the pressure builds up so much that the ear drum perforates or bursts, which instantly relieves the pain. When this happens the outer ear fills up with discharge. Perforations usually heal leaving no damage, but it is advisable for a doctor to check the ear drum a week or so after such a perforation. Infections that do not clear completely, or perforations that do not heal, can cause deafness.

OUTER EAR INFECTION (OTITIS EXTERNA)

The tube leading in from the outer part of the ear up to the ear drum is known as the external auditory meatus (or E.A.M.). It is lined with skin, and this skin can become inflamed and infected, so causing the condition known as otitis externa. Normally this skin remains healthy and doesn't cause problems, but once infection starts it can occasionally be difficult to clear up.

Anything that scratches this very delicate skin can be the trigger for the problem to start. The commonest culprits are cotton buds. Cotton buds are just the ideal size for parents to get them into the ear canal, push any wax in further, and scratch the skin. There is a simple medical law that says 'never put anything into your ear that is smaller than your elbow' and this law applies to parents' and their children's ears equally. (Adults often dig into their ears using paper-clips and ball point pens and this causes just as many problems.)

The other major aggravating factor for otitis externa can be swimming. Whilst middle ear infections tend to happen more in the winter, when they follow colds, outer ear infections are more common in the summer when children swim. Sometimes water – which in some swimming pools, and in particular at hotels in warm countries, may not be perfectly free of infection – can lead to sogginess, inflammation, and infection of the skin of the ear canal.

The pain of otitis externa tends to be different to that of otitis media, and it usually hurts if you tug gently on the ear. The area around the ear can sometimes be slightly tender. The opening of the ear canal may well be swollen, and there is likely to be a greeny, white, or yellow discharge.

CONGESTION OF THE EUSTACHIAN TUBE

Sometimes children, and adults, get earache because the Eustachian canal gets blocked, often when the child has a cold. Normally the air pressure on both sides of the ear drum is equal. It is known that the pressure inside the ear can rise when a child lies down, and if the Eustachian tube is open then this soon equalises. However, when the tube is blocked, the air pressure inside the ear is greater than the pressure outside. The ear drum bulges, and hurts. The answer to this type of problem is more likely to be decongestants than antibiotics, but sometimes the best cure is crying. Crying almost always leads to temporary clearing of the Eustachian tube, and the problem is solved.

PAIN REFERRED FROM THE JAW JOINT

Sometimes children complain of earache, but when the doctor examines the ear he or she can see nothing wrong at all. Occasionally this can be because the problem is actually coming from the jaw joint (otherwise known as the T.M.J. or temporo-mandibular joint). This is relatively unusual in children but much commoner in teenagers and adults. The jaw joint itself, which lies just in front of the ear, may be tender. The usual cause of this problem is dental – perhaps because there might be something wrong with the way the child bites. It is likely your doctor will advise you to consult a dentist.

When to consult a doctor

It is entirely reasonable to seek medical advice if your child complains of earache, but please do give your child paracetamol first. Many is the time that I have been telephoned in the early hours of the morning by parents whose children have earache, and yet who have not given any pain-relieving medication at all. Frequently this is all that you will need to do. There is considerable scientific evidence that most ear infections clear up with simple pain-relieving measures alone, so if you consult the doctor before you have tried giving paracetamol, don't be surprised if the doctor chooses to advise you to give this first.

However, there are a number of reasons why you should consult a doctor *immediately* with a child with earache. These are:

- If your child has a stiff neck (also see 'Meningitis')
- If your child banged his or her head shortly before the earache started
- Your child walks or stands unsteadily, or seems to act 'drunk'
- If your child seems very ill, and has a high fever

In addition, it is entirely reasonable to seek medical help if simple pain-relieving measures are not helping. At the very least, feel free to discuss the situation with a doctor or nurse. Such advice should always be available, if not from your own doctor, then from whoever is covering his or her duties at that time.

How you can help

Earache hurts! The most important first step is to give a full dose of paracetamol. Paracetamol will ease pain, and help to lower any temperature. (See the appendix for full details.) If for any reason your child cannot take paracetamol, then paediatric preparations of ibuprofen should be used.

Earache can also be eased by a warm flannel or hot water bottle held against the ear. However, do take care. Make sure that these are not too hot. Alternatively, if heat actually seems to make things worse, you can try an ice-pack. As long as there is no discharge from the ear (with the risk that there could be a perforated ear drum) you could try putting a couple of drops of warmed olive oil into the ear canal. However, never ever warm the olive oil in a microwave. This can make it surprisingly hot so that you end up with burnt skin in the ear canal, as well as the earache your child started with!

Treatment

Doctors are still undecided as to how important antibiotics are in treating ear infections. In the long-term they don't make much difference, but there is some evidence that pain is relieved sooner if antibiotics are given early.

On the majority of occasions therefore it is likely that your child *will* be given an antibiotic for an ear infection. Children under five will usually be given amoxycillin, erythromycin, or any one of a number of other antibiotics. Over the age of five, penicillin V is the most likely treatment – unless your child is allergic to it. The reason for the different choice at different ages is that the bacteria causing the infection are likely to be different in the older child. It is vitally important to check with your doctor how long the course of treatment should be. Some doctors use very short courses of very high dose antibiotics, whilst most use a longer course of a lower dose. However antibiotics may not be essential, and paracetamol may be all that is needed. And, don't forget, the enormous majority of children grow out of ear infections by the age of six.

Prevention

Children can get a lot of ear infections when they start to go to toddler groups, playgroups, or school but the main reason for this is quite simply because they are more likely to catch colds when they mix with other children. It really does seem to be part of growing up, and to an extent they cannot be completely avoided. However there are two things that do make a difference.

The first is smoking. The children of parents who smoke are much more likely to suffer from ear infections than the children of non-smokers. If you really must smoke, then smoke outside, or away from your child. You owe it to your children. So many childhood conditions are connected with smoking that you owe it to your family to decide that now is the time to stop.

Secondly, there is considerable evidence that bottle-fed children are at a higher risk of developing ear infections than children who are breast-fed.

And remember that with both smoking and bottle-feeding I am simply talking about extra risks. The breast-fed child of a non-smoking family may still get ear infections. It is just less likely to happen as often.

The child with a discharging ear

Symptoms and causes

Several different types of discharge can occur in childhood. Some of these matter, and some of them don't. Whilst you should be able to get a simple idea as to the cause from this section, if you are in any doubt do ask a doctor to have a look.

Yellow, white or green discharge

This is likely to be caused by infection draining out of the ear. The discharge is actually a type of pus, and the infection could be caused by a middle ear infection (otitis media) or an outer ear infection (otitis externa).

Brown or very dark red discharge

This is likely to be wax. Wax is one of the great mysteries of life. Why do some people get so much more than others? Why is it so sticky? If wax is the only ear problem that your child suffers from, as I have said before, there is one golden rule: never ever put anything into your ear that is smaller than your elbow. This may sound a completely absurd statement, but nothing but problems result from things being pushed into the ear. Adults use match-sticks and paperclips. Children get problems from cotton buds. In fact, cotton buds are perfectly designed to push wax further into a child's ear so that it gets compacted inside – just like gunpowder being pushed into a cannon. This makes the wax even harder, and can eventually lead to the ear needing syringing. Simply use cotton buds around the outer ear, but never in the ear canal. Left alone, most wax will clear automatically from the ears. If you try and interfere with this, the chances are you will make things much worse. However, in general, wax really does not matter, unless it is interfering with hearing.

Very occasionally a lot of wax may appear all at once. There is some evidence that this can be caused by an ear infection, with the infection causing a rise in temperature that leads to a slight melting of the wax. This in turn makes it less sticky and it then drains away. If this happens, and in particular if your child has any other signs of an ear infection, then it would be worth asking a doctor to examine the ear. This is not urgent if your child is not ill.

Clear Discharge

If your child has just had his or her hair washed, then a watery discharge is probably just that – water. But if it comes on after any form of head injury, then it is absolutely vital that you see a doctor urgently. A fracture of the base of the skull can lead to cerebro-spinal fluid (the fluid that surrounds the brain) oozing out of the ears. This is rare, but extremely serious.

When to consult a doctor

- If your child has any other evidence of an ear infection
- If the discharge is yellow or pus-y
- If you are concerned about your child's hearing
- If there is a clear discharge that follows a head injury

How you can help

As stated above, never put anything into the ear canal. Simply wipe any discharge clear from the outer part of the ear only, using cotton wool or a cotton bud. Do not use any drops in the ear, just in case there is a perforation. If there is pain, see the section on the child with earache.

Treatment

If the cause is wax, then it is unlikely that anything much will need to be done at all. Wax only needs to be removed if it is causing problems with hearing, but doctors rarely need to arrange for children's ears to be syringed.

If the cause of the discharge is infection, see the section on 'The child with earache' for details of possible treatments.

Prevention

If the cause of the discharge was infection, then you will find full information in the section on 'The child with earache'. However, the single most important thing you can do is keep anything and everything out of the ear. Children who suffer from external ear infections should avoid getting water in the ear, and use ear plugs when swimming.

The child with hearing problems

Hearing really does matter. A child cannot learn to talk properly if he or she cannot hear clearly. The child who cannot hear will be at a disadvantage at playgroup and at school, and when playing with friends. If everything your child hears is muffled, then life can be confusing, and upsetting, and even a little frightening. Most doctors will agree that the most sensitive test for a child's hearing is a parent. If a mother or father says that a child is deaf, then the wise doctor will assume that they are correct – at least until proved otherwise.

Symptoms

Sometimes hearing problems will be all too obvious. If your child doesn't hear you when you say something – particularly if it is words such as 'sweets' or 'do you want an ice-cream?' – then there is likely to be a problem with hearing. The child who does not hear you say 'Tidy your bedroom' is, of course, entirely normal.

An older child may volunteer the information, but it is more likely that a child will not notice when he or she hears less clearly. The change in hearing is usually gradual and taken for granted. However you may get a clue if a child is always shouting, or if the television set is turned up more loudly than usual.

With younger children, the main clue is delay in learning to speak, or even lack of clarity in speech. Later in this section I give some guidelines which should help – but the real message is that if you are in doubt, do have your child checked by your doctor or health visitor.

Causes

On page 74, in the section on 'The child with earache', I describe the normal anatomy of the ear, but in essence there is an outer canal that runs from the outside up to the ear drum. Behind the ear drum there is a cavity, which is connected to the throat by the Eustachian tube. The tiny bones – the hammer, anvil, and stirrup – transmit sound to the inner ear, and the inner ear transmits messages to the brain which are interpreted as sound.

Hearing can be affected if any part of this chain is affected. There are two main forms of deafness, known as conductive deafness and nerve (or perceptive) deafness.

CONDUCTIVE DEAFNESS

In conductive deafness the conduction of sound through the ear is obstructed. This can be with a blockage in the outer ear canal (from wax, or discharge, or even a peanut or bead). The blockage can also be in the middle ear cavity, usually from infection, or glue ear. Glue ear is a type of middle ear infection, in which the fluid in the middle ear cavity is thick and sticky, just like glue. This has the same effect as putting a microphone in a bowl of porridge – sounds are muffled, as the vibrations cannot be passed from the ear drum through the hammer, anvil, and stirrup bones, to the inner ear. There is still uncertainty as to what causes glue ear. Some doctors think it is a result of frequent middle ear infections, but others are less certain. Large adenoids can also block the drainage of the Eustachian tube. Incidentally, the amount of actual fluid in the middle ear cavity may alter considerably from one day to another. If your child seems to hear better on some days than others, then this may be the explanation. It does not mean he or she is having you on!

NERVE DEAFNESS

In nerve deafness the hearing problem lies in the inner ear itself, either in the nerve that sends impulses from the ear to the brain, or within the brain itself. This form of deafness is most typically present from birth, where it can be the result of conditions such as congenital rubella (or German measles). It can also be caused by meningitis, by severe jaundice occurring shortly after birth, by damage occurring during the birth process itself, by some drugs – most of which are rarely used nowadays – and a number of virus infections.

When to consult a doctor

If you are in any doubt about your child's ability to hear, then seek advice. With young children the most valuable pointers to hearing problems are difficulties with speech, and the following guidelines may be helpful in showing when there might be problems in normal development of speech.

If your child fits one of these categories, then do have him or her checked over by your doctor, and, ideally, ask for a hearing test to be performed:

- If your baby is six months old and does not respond consistently to sound
- If your child is one year old and has either not started babbling, or else has started but then stopped
- If you have a toddler who does not use words

- If your two-year-old does not make two-word phrases
- If your two-and-a-half-year-old has speech that is not generally intelligible to you or the family
- If your three-year-old is not making sentences
- If your three-and-a-half-year-old cannot be readily understood by strangers

Hearing problems in babies can be hard to spot, but hearing tests are part of the routine checks for all children in the U.K. The exact timings vary depending on where you live. Clues that deafness may be a problem in babies include:

After birth – the baby not being startled by a loud noise such as a door slamming

By three months – the baby not smiling at the sound of your voice, or turning towards a sound coming from the side

By six months – not turning to your voice or to quiet noises from the side

These tests are obviously very crude, but are enough of a clue for you to be suspicious. If you have any doubts at all, then do please tell your doctor or health visitor. Even the very youngest children can be tested effectively and accurately for hearing problems.

How you can help

The single most important thing that any parent can do about a hearing problem is notice it! There is not an awful lot that can be done in the way of first aid, but if you don't realise that deafness might be the reason why your child shouts, or seems rather slow at school, or is poor at socialising, then really valuable time may be lost.

However, with the simple problem of ear wax, which is a

common cause of deafness, the way you try to deal with it can be vitally important. After all, wax is one of the great mysteries of life. No one really understands why some people get so much more than others, or why it is so sticky, or even why it is there. For answers to these, you will have to look elsewhere. However there is one golden rule of ear-keeping, which I have stated elsewhere in this book as it is so important. Never ever put anything into your child's ear (or even your own ear) that is smaller than your elbow. This may sound a completely absurd statement, but nothing but problems result from things being pushed into the ear. Do not use cotton buds in the ear canal. They are perfectly designed to push wax further into a child's ear so that it gets compacted inside – just like gunpowder being pushed into a cannon. This makes the wax even harder, and can eventually lead to the ear needing syringing. Only use cotton buds around the outer ear. Left alone, most wax will clear automatically from the ears. If you try to interfere with this, the chances are you will make things much worse.

Treatment

The treatment of deafness depends more than anything on what exactly the diagnosis is. The sooner that the diagnosis is made, and treatment is started, the better. With conductive deafness, the treatment will be directed at eliminating whatever is causing the blockage of transmission of sound into the ear. If the cause is wax, this may be gently syringed away by the doctor or nurse, usually after drops such as olive oil have been used to soften the wax first.

Deafness will often result as a temporary problem after a middle ear infection (otitis media) but hearing should normally be back to normal after about three weeks. If a perforation was present and this fails to heal, very occasionally this will need to be repaired surgically in order to restore the hearing.

If the problem is glue ear, or catarrh in the middle ear cavity, the possible treatment is rather more controversial. Frequently the condition gets better by itself if given sufficient time. Other possible treatments might include prolonged courses of antibiotics, decongestants, or even surgery which might be removal of the adenoids, which are like the tonsils and are situated at the lower end of the Eustachian tube, and the insertion of grommets.

Grommets are tiny plastic tubes that are inserted, under an anaesthetic, through a slit made in the ear drum. These allow air to pass into the middle ear cavity, and this allows the pressure in the middle ear cavity to return to normal and be equal with the pressure of the air outside. Recently, some doctors have begun to question how essential this operation really is, though it can be remarkably effective. My own daughter is an example of such a success story. Discuss the need for the operation with your G.P. and specialist before coming to any decision. Incidentally, grommets usually drop out by themselves after a few months, and rarely have to be removed. Most children with grommets are also able to swim, though you need to check about this with your E.N.T. specialist, as it does depend on the type of grommet used.

With perceptive, or nerve deafness, it may be necessary to use a hearing aid. As a parent you may feel upset or disappointed that your child has to use an aid, but the quicker you can help your child adapt to using the aid the better. With severe hearing difficulties you might even need to attend special training in lip reading or signing.

Prevention

Most types of hearing problem cannot be prevented, but do make sure that you are immune to German measles before your next pregnancy. Congenital rubella is a condition that does not need to happen these days.

The child who suffers from repeated ear infections may occasionally be more at risk of long-term hearing difficulties. There is plenty of evidence that children who live in households where someone smokes are more likely to get ear infections than the families of non-smokers. That is yet another reason to give up smoking now.

The child with a stiff, painful or swollen neck

THE CHILD WITH A STIFF OR PAINFUL NECK

Symptoms and causes

A stiff neck can be a sign of meningitis. However vitally important this condition is, the simple fact is that the vast majority of children who complain of a stiff neck do *not* have meningitis, but are instead suffering from some much more minor, benign, condition.

This section is designed to help you begin to discriminate between the different types, but, if in doubt, always consult a doctor.

In meningitis, the stiffness prevents the child being able to bend the head forward. The muscles in the back of the neck are affected, and you can best test for this in a toddler by lying them down, and asking them to look at his or her tummy button. This will make the child bend the head slightly forward, and if your child can do this, then meningitis is extremely unlikely. In older children, you can ask them to put their chin onto their chest. Meningitis is almost always associated with severe headache and a raised temperature.

However, as I have already mentioned, whilst meningitis is the most important cause of a stiff neck, it is by far the least likely. It is very common for children, and adults, to develop a spasm in one side of the neck, either after a minor injury, or on waking up in the morning. This last condition is called a 'wry neck', and the child will find it difficult to move his or her head from side to side, which is best shown by asking the child to put his or her chin on each shoulder in turn. In wry neck this will be possible on one side, but not on the other. Moving the chin onto the chest is typically painless, and the child will be well in every other way.

Treatment

In this condition, one of the most effective treatments is either a warm hot water bottle held onto the area of spasm for a couple of minutes every hour (but make sure it is only comfortably warm!), or alternatively an ice-pack. Take a small bag of frozen peas or sweet corn, wrap it in a tea towel, and hold this against the affected area instead – then gently encourage your child to move the neck. Using paracetamol of ibuprofen can be beneficial too.

When to consult a doctor

If the discomfort is severe, or lasts more than twenty-four hours, see your doctor who might need to arrange physiotherapy.

THE CHILD WITH A SWOLLEN NECK

A swollen neck may take two main forms. You may notice one or more swellings in your child's neck in a number of different places, or there may possibly be a large diffuse swelling across most of the front of the neck. Most causes of swelling in the neck are entirely harmless, but there are a number of very serious problems that can present in this way. It is therefore absolutely essential that you do not ignore a potentially serious cause. This section should help you begin to unravel the different possibilities, but in doubt seek medical advice.

Symptoms and causes

In children it is very common to detect glands in the neck and around the back of the head from time to time. You may come across these almost by accident, perhaps when dressing your child and doing up the top button, or when combing your child's hair.

The glands that you can feel are lymph nodes. These are scattered all over the body, and as well as being in the neck can be found in the armpits, in the groin, and around the elbows, as well as in a number of other places. Lymph nodes are part of the body's natural defence mechanism, and swell up in the presence of infection to prevent the infection spreading further into the body. For instance, when you or your child has a sore throat, the cervical glands in the front of the neck will be likely to swell, and so prevent the infection spreading onto the chest. As you know, children get a very large number of sore throats and other upper respiratory infections, and the glands are very frequently swollen, even between attacks.

Glands at the back of the neck and behind the ears tend to swell up with certain virus infections, such as German measles or roseola infantum, and also with chickenpox. Infected eczema, or other skin conditions, on the scalp can also lead to swelling of the glands at the back of the neck. Children sometimes complain of neck discomfort if they have swollen glands which result from a throat infection. The swelling will typically be on just one side.

If your child has one of these infections, with perhaps a raised temperature, then you rarely have to be concerned about the swollen glands. They should disappear at the end of the infection. These glands will typically move under your fingers, and whilst being quite firm are not actually woody or rock hard, or stuck to each other. If your child does have a number of very hard glands which are rock hard and are stuck together, then you should very definitely seek medical advice.

When to consult a doctor

Sometimes, however, your child may develop swollen glands without any sign of infection. These, too, will usually disappear over a couple of weeks. If they don't, or if they seem to be enlarging, or if you are concerned that your child is less well than usual, or if you are just plain worried, then do seek your doctor's advice and assessment. If at any stage your child has glands that are either hot or tender, then do see a doctor right away. It is likely that your child will need antibiotics.

So – in summary – do consult your doctor if any lumps in the neck persist for longer than three weeks, or if any of them are either very large, very tender, or are red.

If the swelling in the neck is more central, and in particular if it moves upwards when your child swallows, this could possibly be a swelling in the thyroid gland – the gland that controls the body's metabolism. An overactive thyroid would, generally, make your child overactive, always on the go, possibly lose weight, and have a rapid heart beat. An underactive gland, by contrast, causes sluggishness. A sufferer generally will be slowed down, with dry hair, dry skin, constipation, and a slow pulse rate. These conditions are both unusual in children, but to check up on this it really is important that you consult a doctor.

The child with a headache

Symptoms

Headaches cause tremendous anxiety for parents. On the one hand we know that in adults they can be tremendously common. Indeed we all suffer from headaches from time to time. But if a child gets a headache, most parents' thoughts turn immediately to meningitis – one of every parent's worst fears. This chapter will help to unravel the different types of headache, and on page 100 give a clear and authoritative guide as to when you should seek urgent medical attention.

The main symptom of headache is, of course, headache. Hardly worth saying. But beware, sometimes when children talk about a headache they may not be referring to a pain in the head. I remember asking a four-year-old where she felt her headache, and she pointed at her tummy. Other children talk about 'headaches' when they simply feel unhappy or fed up – something they might copy from an adult who keeps complaining about everything being a headache.

Headaches are actually remarkably common in children. Estimates suggest that nearly a quarter of primary schoolchildren and nearly nine out of ten secondary schoolchildren suffer occasional headaches, and probably one child in ten suffers from migraine. Nevertheless there are still parents, and doctors, who think this is rare. In addition, depending on the type of headache, there may be other symptoms. For instance, the child with migraine may also have nausea.

Causes

With most headaches – certainly in adults and older children – the chances are that you will never find a cause. I am sure that you have had days when you have perhaps been very stressed and have ended up with a pounding headache. I am also sure that you will accept that the most thorough doctor would not be able to find anything physically wrong with your head, however carefully he or she examined you. This doesn't mean that there is nothing wrong – the pounding pain makes that all too clear and is certainly not imaginary – but physical causes may be very hard to come by.

There are many different types of headache, and I will discuss these one by one. Each type can hurt every bit as much as any other form.

Simple headaches

These are very common, can be very painful, and can be caused by virus infections, fever, not drinking enough, or tiredness. Very occasionally a particular food may be the culprit (in adults the Chinese restaurant syndrome is the most marked and is caused by a sensitivity to monosodium glutamate). Incidentally 'eye strain', which is often blamed for headache, is actually extremely rare.

Tension headaches

These are probably the commonest form of childhood headache, and can be caused by almost any form of upset, tension, or excitement. They can be about school, bullying, homework, shyness, holidays, Christmas, or almost anything else. Indeed frequently it will be a combination of these that cause the headaches. The pain of tension headaches is felt mainly either at the front, or as a band round the head. Both sides of the head tend to be affected equally and at the same time.

Migraine

This type of headache is usually one-sided. The word 'migraine' comes from the Latin words 'hemi' meaning half and 'cranium' meaning head. 'Hemicranium' gets shortened to 'migraine', which also gives a guidance as to how this word should be pronounced. Contrary to what many people say, it should be 'Me Grain' not 'My Grain'! It is becoming clear that many children with frequent headaches are suffering from a form of migraine, even if they don't have all these typical symptoms. Indeed, one could even say that the typical symptoms of adult migraine are unusual in childhood!

Migraine typically runs in families, and there will almost always be a relative with migraine. Typically associated with nausea, tummy ache or vomiting. Some children have recurrent tummy aches occurring occasionally for months or years before the headaches start.

The migraine headache itself may start with visual symptoms such as spots in eyes, zig zag lines, or even a sensation that part of the area of vision is missing. There can also be a temporary numbness or pins and needles in an arm or leg, again coming on primarily before the headache.

Meningitis

Meningitis is an infection of the meninges, the membranes that cover the brain and spinal cord.

There are two main types – those caused by viruses, and

those caused by bacteria – though it takes hospital tests to distinguish between these. Viral meningitis almost always results in a full recovery. Bacterial meningitis, particularly meningitis caused by the bacterium known as the meningococcus, may be fatal. Meningitis is a medical emergency. Overall, less than one child in twenty with meningitis will die – but one in twenty is a high enough figure. Meningitis can also leave disabilities such as severe deafness, epilepsy, or cerebral palsy.

Typically the child has other symptoms before the headache starts. These may be as mild as a sore throat and fever. A child with these symptoms who then develops severe headache and vomiting, and especially if a rash develops, should be seen urgently by a doctor. Either call your G.P. or go immediately to your local hospital – assuming that it has an emergency department. These days not all hospitals do have medical staff available for emergencies. If in doubt, phone 999.

Sinusitis

The sinuses are air-filled cavities lined with mucous membrane in the bones surrounding the nose. Infection can spread to the sinuses from the nose. When this happens, the membranes swell and this blocks the drainage between the sinus and the nose. Pus then builds up in the sinus causing headache. It usually responds well to antibiotics.

Sinusitis can cause headaches in older children, but is not a common problem. This is largely because the sinuses are nowhere near as developed in children as they are in adults.

Brain Tumours

The thought of brain tumours terrifies all parents, but they are extremely rare, affecting only 0.005 per cent of all children. Other symptoms that may be caused by brain tumours include convulsion, behavioural change, muscle weakness, visual changes, and difficulties with speech. All of these are caused by increasing pressure within the skull caused by the tumour.

Other causes

These can include an after effect of a head injury, depression (which is certainly not unheard of in children) and carbon monoxide poisoning. If everyone in the household is suffering from headaches, and you use gas for cooking or heating, then a gas leak can be a possible cause.

When to consult a doctor

There are two reasons to consult a doctor – for sudden very severe headaches, and for less severe headaches that keep returning, or never completely go away, although the longer a child has had headaches, and the longer they last, in general the less likely they are to have a serious cause.

Sudden headaches

Consult a doctor IMMEDIATELY if your child has any of the following:

- Headache following a head injury
- Confusion, unusual behaviour
- Vomiting more than once
- A stiff neck

- Severe pain – a child who screams with pain
- Pain which gets worse despite paracetamol
- Headache that lasts more than twelve hours
- A reluctance to be moved
- An aversion to light
- Blurred vision

RECURRENT HEADACHES

If your child keeps suffering from headaches, which may or may not be migraine, then do consult your doctor to get a definite diagnosis, and to look into the various methods that can be used to prevent the headaches. Migraines can sometimes be prevented by dietary adjustment, by careful calculation of what the causes might be and taking action to sort these out, or by the use of preventative drugs such as pizotifen (Sanomigran) or beta blockers.

In addition, always consult your doctor if:

- The headaches mean your child is frequently missing school
- The pain is usually one-sided
- Your child seems in any other way to be unwell
- The headaches are worse in the morning
- You have a child aged under five who keeps getting headaches

How you can help

Reassurance and dealing with any anxieties and fears is extremely important. In addition, distraction – and every parent knows how best to take their child's mind off things – can be helpful for mild headaches.

Treatment

For most children the most important medication that can help to ease the pain of headaches is paracetamol – but it is important to give it early enough. It seems likely that it is less effective for headaches that have already taken a hold.

Prevention

Prevention can certainly be important in migraine. For other types of headaches prevention is obviously only possible if you can work out what might be causing them. A tension headache caused by bullying is, of course, best treated by tackling the bullying – but what is best is not always easiest!

In migraine, if they are very frequent, it is possible to use prophylactic – preventative – medication in older children. In addition, you should talk to your doctor about using a symptom diary to see if you can work out what the trigger might be. Such things as foods (particularly chocolate), hunger, tiredness, stress, and so on can all be relevant. However food triggers are all or nothing. The food either causes migraine or it doesn't, so there is no need to ban chocolate from your child's life, if you know that he or she can eat chocolate without getting a migraine.

Meningitis – every parent's fear

Symptoms in infants

Early

- Drowsiness
- Irritability
- Off feeds
- Distress on handling

- Vomiting or diarrhoea
- Fever

More specific symptoms

- Neck stiffness
- Tense or bulging fontanelle (the 'soft spot' in the skull)
- A purple (bruise-like) rash that does not disappear when you press it. A simple test is to press a glass drinking tumbler against the rash with the glass against the skin. In meningitis the rash will not fade but remains visible through the glass

Late symptoms

- High-pitched or moaning cry
- Coma
- Shock
- A widespread and rapidly spreading purple rash

Symptoms in older children

Early

- Vomiting
- Fever
- Headache
- Back or joint pains

More specific symptoms

- Neck stiffness
- Aversion to bright light
- A purple (bruise-like) rash that does not disappear when you press it
- Confusion

Late symptoms

- Coma
- Shock
- A widespread and rapidly spreading purple rash

If you suspect that your child might have meningitis seek medical attention NOW. Either take your child immediately to a casualty unit, dial 999 for an ambulance, or call your G.P. Take whichever action will be the quickest to get your child seen by a doctor. In this condition minutes count.

The child with nose problems

This chapter will look at some very common problems that can affect children's noses. The main topics under consideration are:

- Nose bleeds
- Nasal congestion
- Snoring and mouth breathing
- Foreign bodies in the nose
- Sneezing
- Sniffing

The subject of hayfever is dealt with fully in the chapter on 'The child with allergies'.

NOSE BLEEDS

These are often truly dramatic, and very frightening. It can sometimes look as if your child has bled pints and pints of blood. In the far-off days when I was a medical student, before there was concern about H.I.V. and similar infections, I remember a dramatic demonstration by one of our lecturers. A colleague sat in a plastic mac on a plastic sheet, and the lecturer poured a pint of blood over her! 'That', he said, 'is what a pint of blood looks like!' It seemed to go everywhere. 'When patients tell you that they've bled a pint or more, you will now know whether their estimate is true or not.' It was an extraordinary demonstration, but it taught me that a little blood can go a very long way. Your child may look as if he or she has bled a pint, but it is probably more like a tea-cup full.

Causes

It is extremely uncommon indeed for nose bleeds in children to be caused by high blood pressure. Some children do seem to have more nose bleeds than others for no very good reason, but if your child has repeated bleeds then do see your doctor to make sure that there is not a problem with the way his or her blood clots.

Perhaps the most frequent cause of childhood nose bleeds is nose-picking. The finger that is surreptitiously inserted for a good pick is the best way to get bleeding to start again!

Finally, nasal congestion can sometimes make the lining of the nose more fragile, so triggering off nose bleeds. This is dealt with later in this section.

Treatment

Countless myths and old wives tales surround nose bleeds. Suggested treatments include dangling a cold key down the back of the neck – though how this is supposed to work I have no idea. In fact, the treatment for a heavy nose bleed is usually quite straightforward:

- Sit the child up, so that his or her head is over a bowl. This way any bleeding will come out of the nose rather than down the back of the throat.
- Squeeze the bridge of the nose firmly for five minutes. Use a watch. Without accurate timing, you will probably think that five minutes are up when actually only two minutes have passed. Don't be tempted to have a look to see if bleeding has stopped before the five minutes are up.
- If the bleeding is very heavy, put a couple of ice cubes in a polythene bag, and squeeze the nose between these for five minutes.

- Once the bleeding has stopped, do not let your child blow his nose for at least half an hour – and then only gently. Don't worry if there is a large blood clot just inside the nostril. Blowing will dislodge this and set the bleeding going again.
- If this treatment doesn't do the trick, then the bleeding blood vessel in the nose will probably need cauterising. Contact your doctor's practice. Some practices are able to do this. Others will advise you to go to your local hospital.

Don't panic if your child vomits blood after a nose bleed. Blood that is swallowed can often be vomited back up, and this does not make the problem any more serious.

Don't ever try and pack the nose with cotton wool or gauze. It's unlikely to work, and it may well get stuck!

NASAL CONGESTION

The nose, sinuses, throat, ears and mouth are all interconnected, and problems affecting any one of these can spread to another. Infections are particularly common in children, who can sometimes seem to get one cold after another.

The nose itself is lined with fine tissue called mucous membrane, and this can become inflamed and swell up in a number of conditions. The effect of this will either be blocking of the nose, or a runny nose. In addition, there is a bone running down the centre of the nose called the nasal septum. This should be absolutely central, and if for any reason it is displaced to one side, this too can lead to blockage of the nose. The commonest cause for a deviated nasal septum is an injury to the nose.

Causes

By far the commonest cause of nasal congestion is 'allergic rhinitis'. There are two main forms of this: 'seasonal rhinitis', otherwise known as hayfever, and 'perennial rhinitis', the equivalent of hayfever that lasts all year round. Allergic rhinitis tends to run in families, and is generally commoner in teenagers than younger children. It can be triggered by allergy to almost anything that is present year round, but the most common triggers are house-dust or house-dust mites, animals, birds, moulds, chemicals, or plants, although sometimes no obvious cause can be found. Allergic rhinitis is dealt with in a great deal of detail in the section on hayfever on page 240.

The other common cause of congestion is catarrh – which is an accumulation of mucus at the back of the nose and throat. If there is a nasal discharge that is green or yellow this frequently means that there is a bacterial infection of the nose or sinuses. However, if there is a green or yellow discharge from just one side of the nose, then this makes it extremely likely that your child has stuck a small object up the nose. This could be a bead, or a nut, or suchlike.

Treatment

Never attempt to get a foreign body out yourself. Always see a doctor. Infection may well need antibiotics.

SNORING AND MOUTH BREATHING

Causes

Mouth breathing is particularly common in children aged four to five years. This is due to a combination of factors. Both the tonsils and the adenoids (glandular swellings found at the back of the nasal passage above the tonsils) are at their largest, and these may block the space at the back of the nose. If the nose is blocked, the child inevitably has to breathe through his or her mouth. The blockage can also cause night-time snoring, which can reach a remarkable decibel level. Snoring and mouth breathing can also be aggravated by any of the conditions that can cause nasal congestion and which I describe above.

Treatment

There are many curious traditional remedies for snoring, such as sewing a cork into the back of the pyjamas or nightie to stop the sufferer sleeping on his or her back. Please don't try any of these with a small child. If the snoring continues, you should always consult a doctor to have the cause correctly diagnosed. Severe snoring can sometimes interfere with the quality of sleep and cause daytime tiredness, so it is certainly not a matter to be dismissed lightly. Treatment can involve decongestants, nasal sprays or drops, or even ocasionally surgery.

FOREIGN BODIES IN THE NOSE

Causes

Some small children have a terrible habit of pushing tiny objects into almost any available bodily orifice, and the nostrils are one of the most easily accessible. Beads, peanuts, sweets, and tiny Lego bricks are just some of the foreign bodies that I have had to extract from young noses over the years.

Treatment

If you know for certain that your child has definitely pushed something up his or her nose, contact your doctor for advice. In general these problems are best handled at hospital, but some general practices have the facilities for successfully extracting these delights. Speak to the practice on the phone first to determine what you should do.

However, not every nasal foreign body is so easy to identify. A common enough scenario is for the child to develop a foul-smelling green or yellow nasal discharge from just one side of the nose. If this happens, it usually means that a foreign body has been inserted and forgotten. Blowing the nose is unlikely to be helpful. Go and seek your doctor's help. Incidentally, if your child makes a habit of repeatedly inserting objects into any bodily orifice, then your doctor needs to know about this as well. It can be a sign of a psychological problem, and the sooner this is picked up and acted on the better.

SNEEZING

Causes

Occasional sneezing is normal. It is the body's highly efficient way of expelling irritants from inside the nose, and jettisons pollen or pepper at high speed and with great force.

Treatment

The child who repeatedly sneezes is likely to have a form of allergic rhinitis, such as hayfever, and this is covered in depth on page 243.

SNIFFING

Causes

The child who has recently started sniffing will be likely to have a cold, although some children then seem to go on and on sniffing repeatedly even after the cold gets better. It is likely that this will be a matter of habit, but sometimes there may be an underlying problem such as enlarged adenoids or allergic rhinitis. I would therefore recommend that your child should be checked over by the doctor.

Treatment

The best cure for sniffing involves teaching your child to blow his or her nose properly. However, as little boys in particular seem congenitally unable to know how to use a handkerchief, this can be harder than it sounds!

The child with mouth problems

This chapter deals with three problems:
• Mouth ulcers
• Geographical tongue
• Tongue tie

MOUTH ULCERS

Symptoms

Mouth ulcers are open sores that are caused by a tiny break in the mucous membrane, the soft pink tissue that lines the mouth. This is, incidentally, the same type of tissue that also lines the respiratory tract, gut, urinary and genital systems, and even the eyelids. It is known as mucous membrane as it secretes mucous, a fluid which keeps all these structures moist and well lubricated.

Typically, mouth ulcers are round or oval spots which may be white, yellow, or even grey, sometimes you will see one by itself, or there may possibly be a cluster. And they hurt!

The two main types of mouth ulcer are:

Apthous ulcers
Herpes simplex ulcers

In addition, children may also develop mouth ulcers if they are suffering from hand, foot, and mouth disease – see page 211.

Causes

Apthous ulcers can occur at any age, although they are most common in children over the age of ten years. Without treatment they typically last up to about two weeks. There are a number of possible causes. Trauma to the lining of the mouth is a common trigger. The trauma may be due to careless use of a toothbrush or from the child putting his fingers (and hence fingernails) in his mouth. Sometimes these ulcers are associated with infection with the streptococcus bacteria, which frequently cause throat infections. They are also more common in children with a family history of recurrent apthous ulcers.

Apthous ulcers can also be associated with various types of anaemia and some children and adults develop ulcers if they eat particular foods, with this almost certainly being a genuine form of food intolerance. Particularly troublesome may be nuts, tomatoes, and wheat products.

Herpes simplex ulcers are caused by the herpes simplex virus which also causes cold sores. Cold sores typically appear on the outside edge of the lips. If this is the cause of the ulcers, your child would be likely also to have a raised temperature and swollen glands in the neck, and may feel generally unwell.

When to consult a doctor

The occasional mouth ulcer is just a nuisance, and probably only needs the simple self-help measures outlined below. If your child keeps having these ulcers, however, you should consult your doctor for further advice, and also to find out if there is any underlying cause, such as anaemia.

If your child has any of the signs of herpes mouth ulceration that I have described above, do consult your doctor for assessment, advice, and treatment.

Treatment

Most mouth ulcers cure themselves without needing any particular treatment, but the pain can be eased by using analgesic mouth gels or mouth washes. Your pharmacist should be able to advise you about these. Large ulcers, or ulcers that are slow to disappear, may be helped by steroid tablets that should be dissolved against the ulcer, or steroid pastes (such as Adcortyl in Orabase) which can be applied to the ulcer, and which stick remarkably firmly. These may be prescribed by your doctor.

Prevention

If your child is a habitual finger chewer, then discouraging this practice may well be helpful. Apart from this, mouth ulcers are particularly difficult to prevent, unless you or your doctor can detect an underlying cause or trigger factor.

GEOGRAPHICAL TONGUE

The tongue consists of a mass of muscle, covered by mucous membrane. The surface of the tongue is naturally rough, with tiny nodules called papillae that project from the upper surface. At the back of the tongue are the vallate papillae, much larger, round elevated projections that parents sometimes see for the first time and are understandably concerned about. However, these are entirely normal.

In the condition known as geographical tongue, areas of the tongue appear smooth and flattened, often with an elevated grey rim. The name comes from the fact that these flat patches look like continents on a map, lying in the sea.

Geographical tongue is completely painless and does not affect either taste or any other tongue function. Occasionally, it may be linked with psoriasis, virus infections, or overuse of mouthwashes, but in the vast majority of cases no cause is found. It simply disappears by itself after weeks, months, or (occasionally) years, leaving no after effects at all. The best solution to worrying about what the tongue looks like is not to look at it!

TONGUE TIE

Running from the undersurface of the tongue is a band of tissue that connects the tongue to the floor of the mouth. If you gently feel under your own tongue you will find it very easily. This tissue is known as the frenulum, and in the condition of tongue tie the frenulum is short and tight, so preventing easy movement of the tongue. Theoretically, this could also interfere with speech, and in the past many children had a tongue tie divided as parents and doctors worried that normal speech development was being impaired.

In fact, genuine tongue tie that needs medical attention is incredibly rare. In very many years as a G.P., I can only think of a couple of children who needed the frenulum dividing. Nevertheless, huge numbers of parents have brought their children to see me, worried that their baby has tongue tie, a fear often triggered by the comments of well-meaning relatives. A degree of tongue tie is normal in babies and does not cause any problems at all. If you are still worried, do have a word with your doctor. He or she will soon be able to put your mind at rest. Obviously, any operation to loosen the frenulum should be avoided unless it is absolutely essential.

The child with toothache

Symptoms

Few adults will have escaped the pain of toothache. It can be one of the most irritating, frustrating, dispiriting pains imaginable – enough to drive you to extraction. Our children, however, seem generally to be having a better time of it. Fluoride toothpaste, less aggressive dentistry, and generally improved dental hygiene all seem to have greatly reduced the incidence of dental caries (decay) in children. I have a mouth full of fillings, but both my son and daughter managed to get through childhood without needing a single filling – and our experience is quite typical.

Nevertheless, children do still occasionally suffer painful teeth, and, whilst they are teething, small babies can obviously have a thoroughly miserable time.

Causes

TEETHING

Most babies suffer discomfort while their teeth are erupting, and, when you consider what is happening, it is really little wonder! Teeth begin to develop well before they actually appear in the mouth, with the initial stages happening before birth – and a few babies actually being born with one or more teeth already showing. The first teeth to appear are the incisors – the teeth at the very front of the mouth – followed by the molars (at the back), and then the canines (between the incisors and molars). Typically, the twenty primary teeth will have appeared by the age of two and a half years.

At the age of about six years, the permanent teeth begin to appear, starting this time with the molars. The full set of permanent teeth (with the exception of the wisdom teeth) will have appeared by the start of the teenage years.

Despite what many people believe, there is no evidence that problems such as diarrhoea, rashes, or coughs are associated with teething. The only things that teething causes are dribbling, discomfort, and teeth. These other problems are just common at the same age.

As the tooth is coming through, the gum over the emerging tooth is typically red and inflamed, and sometimes a blister may cover the tooth as it first pokes through the surface of the gum.

TOOTH DECAY

Apart from teething, the other prime cause of toothache in children is tooth decay. Otherwise known as dental caries, this is typically associated with poor dental hygiene and eating sugary foods frequently. The first step in dental decay is the formation of plaque, which is a deposit on the teeth made from food particles, saliva, and bacteria. The combination of plaque and sugar leads to the formation of acid which wears away at the dental enamel covering the tooth. Initially, the decay affects just the enamel covering the tooth. It then moves on to the dentine, the material which makes up the bulk of the tooth. Eventually, even the inner core of the tooth, the pulp, may be affected. Primary teeth are no more prone to tooth decay than the later teeth, but because they are smaller and have relatively larger pulps, the decay appears to occur much more rapidly. Sometimes the first teeth may appear to be decaying almost as soon as they erupt, and this is particularly a problem in children who have a lot of exposure to sugar, especially in the form of sweetened dummies.

When to consult a doctor

With simple teething, it is unlikely that you will need to seek medical or dental help unless the problem is unusually severe and simple measures (as described below) don't do the trick. However, with toothache in a child who is not teething, I believe you should always seek a dentist's advice. You can use pain killers while you are waiting, but toothache should never be ignored. (Incidentally, if a child injures or damages a tooth, you should also seek dental help straight away. If a tooth is knocked out, rinse it in cooled boiled water and try to insert it back into the socket if you possibly can while you go straight to the dentist, or dental hospital.)

In a child with a gum boil, which is the old term for a dental abscess, you might choose to consult your doctor initially as antibiotics may be necessary, but he or she is also likely to advise you to consult the dentist for a more detailed assessment. A dental abscess consists of a pus-filled sac in the tissue around the root of a tooth, and typically causes the affected tooth to ache or throb. The gum around the tooth is particularly tender, and the boil may burst, discharging foul-tasting pus into the mouth. You should never ignore a dental abscess, or simply give your child your G.P.'s antibiotics and fail to follow it up when it seems to feel better. Without further assessment, the problem is likely to recur.

Treatment

The baby who is teething may well be irritable and miserable. Some babies find that chewing on a hard, smooth object like a teething ring, a dried crust of bread, or a scrubbed carrot, can help. Don't leave your baby alone with any of these in case he or she chokes. Rusks are acceptable as teething aids if you can find one that is genuinely sugar-free. Paracetamol can also be helpful, and for babies aged over four months you might try some of the teething gels that you will find at your chemist's, but do avoid teething gels that contain aspirin, and preferably choose one that is sugar-free.

Treat the older child who has toothache with paracetamol or ibuprofen until you are able to consult your dentist.

Prevention

There is no way of preventing the pain of teething. However, dental caries is very definitely preventable. The main secret is careful and regular brushing, the use of fluoride toothpaste, and avoiding too many sugary foods. Sugary bedtime drinks in particular should be avoided, unless you can ensure that the teeth are thoroughly cleaned afterwards. Brush your child's teeth and gums thoroughly twice each day. You should use no more than a pea-sized amount of fluoride toothpaste, as too much fluoride can actually cause problems in itself.

Register your baby with a dentist as soon as you can after birth, and remember that NHS dental care is free for children. You really should talk to your dentist or dental hygienist about the most appropriate measures to take to keep your child's teeth as healthy as possible. In some areas, fluoride supplements may be useful. In addition, some dentists may offer fissure sealing, or other techniques.

The child who vomits

Symptoms

Vomiting can either occur by itself, or very frequently it happens in association with diarrhoea. A full description of conditions such as gastroenteritis, which cause diarrhoea and vomiting ('D&V') is given in the section on 'The child with diarrhoea'.

It is normal for babies to regurgitate, or posset, their food and this can occur for many reasons. The difference between simple posseting and full-blown vomiting can sometimes be difficult to distinguish. However, in vomiting there is more force to the ejection of the contents of the stomach, typically milk. In posseting the milk simply dribbles out of the mouth.

VOMITING IN SMALL BABIES

Causes

Pyloric stenosis

The most important cause of forceful vomiting in babies is a condition known as pyloric stenosis. In this problem, there is thickening of the pylorus, the strong muscular valve at the point where the stomach empties into the duodenum, and this results in little in the way of stomach contents being able to get past it. As milk is taken into the stomach, it is unable to pass into the rest of the gut. The stomach muscle tightens in an attempt to force the gastric contents past the blockage, and as this cannot happen the stomach contents are then ejected forcefully up through the oesophagus and out. This is known as projectile vomiting, and the curdled milk positively shoots out of the mouth.

Pyloric stenosis tends to run in families, and is four times as common in males as in females.

Occasional projectile vomiting is not uncommon, but if it happens repeatedly you should certainly consult a doctor. Pyloric stenosis usually causes symptoms at between two and six weeks of age, and babies with this condition are typically hungry, crying to be fed almost immediately after the vomit. The hunger is simply a result of the lack of food being able to get into the intestine for normal absorption. The vomit is never stained with the yellow-green colour of bile, because bile is added to the gut contents after the pylorus. Babies with this condition are also constipated, and fail to gain weight.

If your doctor suspects pyloric stenosis then your baby will be admitted to hospital. Initially this will be for observation, and possibly a scan, but when the diagnosis has been made there is only one effective treatment and that is surgery. The operation, known as Ramstedt's operation, is now routine and extremely safe. It involves dividing some of the muscle fibres at the pylorus, so relieving the obstruction. It usually leaves a relatively tiny scar, and no after effects whatsoever.

Other causes

Some babies vomit more with one type of milk formula than another, and vomiting is one of the few good reasons to experiment with a change in type of milk formula. Infants who vomit repeatedly in the first few days of life must be assessed by a doctor, as this could be a sign of some form of bowel obstruction, or possibly an infection.

VOMITING AT OTHER AGES

At any age, sudden onset vomiting is most likely to be linked with some sort of infection. This could be a gut infection (gastroenteritis) but could equally likely be almost any other infection – including throat, chest, or ear infections, urine infections, or even more serious conditions such as meningitis. When the cause is an infection the child will almost always have a raised temperature, and other symptoms which should help to pinpoint the cause of the sickness. If in doubt, seek medical advice.

As well as being part of D&V, vomiting can also occur as part of another illness. Almost anything may start it, from a simple cold, to tonsillitis, ear infections, and so on. Vomiting can also be associated with other conditions like meningitis, but there are obviously usually other signs of illness as well. The combination of abdominal pain and vomiting should always lead you to seek medical advice. The commonest cause is likely to be gastroenteritis, which tends to cause colicky crampy pains that come and go.

One other common reason for vomiting is travel sickness. With luck, you should be able to avoid this when travelling by car by ensuring that your child can see out of the window, using a booster seat if necessary. In addition try to ensure that he or she does not spend the journey looking down at toys or books, and by avoiding large meals or drinks before the journey. Small dry snacks, such as biscuits, are also helpful, as are sweets which can be sucked. Distractions in the form of stories or songs on cassette tapes can help a great deal – but if all else fails, have a word with your doctor or pharmacist about suitable travel sickness medication.

When to consult a doctor

Simple vomiting, caused by a gastric upset, does not usually last for much more than six to eight hours. If a baby is sick for longer than this, ask your doctor's advice. You should generally ask sooner if your baby also has diarrhoea. If an older child does not keep drinks down after twelve hours then you should also seek help.

The most important problem to look out for is any sign of dehydration. The child who is dehydrated tends to be listless and tired, and has a dry tongue. The skin lacks elasticity, something that you can judge by squeezing a fold of skin, either over the front of the abdomen or back of the hand, between your finger and thumb, and then letting go. The skin should spring back to its normal appearance immediately. If it only returns to normal slowly, then your child may be too dry, and you should seek medical help.

In addition, a child who is dehydrated will pass much less urine than normal. Indeed, dehydration is likely if no urine has been passed for six hours. The best way to judge a dry tongue is by washing your hands and then putting a clean finger in to your baby's mouth. The tongue and mouth don't normally feel dry, but if your child is dehydrated then they might. In babies, the fontanelle (soft spot) on the top of the head may be sunken in dehydration.

Vomiting with a headache, particularly if the child also has a temperature, could possibly be meningitis. Don't hesitate to seek medical help, although it is far more likely to be something much less serious like a throat infection.

Blood in the vomit is not uncommon, and is usually harmless, but nevertheless I believe your child should always be assessed by a doctor if this happens. The commonest cause is repeated retching and heaving, probably caused by a simple tummy bug, which then leads to slight tearing of the lining of the stomach or lower oesophagus.

Another very common cause of blood in the vomit is a nose bleed. Some children with a nose bleed will swallow the blood, and then may vomit this very dark blood up some time later. The appearance of blood in this way can be enormously frightening.

How you can help

When treating a vomiting child, remember that small sips of fluid are easier to keep down than larger quantities of drink. Coca Cola, or similar drinks, also seem to stay down more easily, but are best given flat rather than fizzy. These drinks are available almost everywhere in the world, so can solve your treatment problems if you are away on holiday. However, even better than these are proprietary treatments for diarrhoea and vomiting such as Rehidrat or Dioralyte sachets. When using these – or any other form of drinks – wait a while after a spell of vomiting before offering more drink. If you give a drink straight after a vomit, it is almost bound to come back up.

Treatment

As mentioned above, the mainstay of treatment is fluid replacement. You can either purchase a suitable product, or be prescribed it by your doctor. Ideally you should use properly formulated electrolyte mixtures such as Rehidrat, Dioralyte, and such-like. Drugs are very rarely used in children to control vomiting. The side effects can be worse than the condition itself.

If your baby is being breast-fed and starts to vomit, then it is perfectly all right – and indeed wise – to continue giving breast milk.

As far as eating and drinking are concerned, I discuss this at some length in the section on diarrhoea, but in essence I believe that you should let your child be the guide. Offer food and drink when he or she asks – but initially it is best to start with clear fluids. If tummy ache causes pain, you can always give paracetamol.

Prevention

If there is an epidemic of gastroenteritis, then the most important aspect of prevention is hygiene. This is vitally important. Regularly washing your hands, particularly after going to the toilet, is essential for every member of the family. Sad to say, it is not always effective – though this doesn't make it any less important.

Here is a summary of when to consult a doctor:

- Vomiting with any sign of dehydration
- Persistent projectile vomiting
- Vomiting with headache or neck stiffness
- Vomiting with severe abdominal pain
- Blood in the vomit
- Vomiting coming on after a head injury
- If your child's abdomen appears hard, or swollen, or seems tender when you touch it
- Vomiting in a child who appears ill
- Vomiting in a baby for more than six hours
- Vomiting in an older child for more than twelve hours
- If your child vomits even when he or she has not taken any food or drink by mouth

The child with diarrhoea

Symptoms

Diarrhoea simply means a change in the pattern of bowel motions with watery and more frequent stools. It is this change in pattern that is important. Breast-fed infants may have half a dozen fairly loose stools each and every day, but this does not mean they have diarrhoea. Indeed, children vary widely in how often they go to the loo.

Causes

Before explaining the many possible causes of diarrhoea, it would be sensible to run through a brief summary of the normal anatomy and working of the bowel. Food initially enters the stomach, where it is mixed with acids and other digestive juices, and the powerful muscular walls of the stomach help to pulp it. The food then passes through a valve, the pyloric sphincter, into the small intestine. Here further enzymes in the digestive juices help to break the food down even further and the rhythmic contractions of the bowel help to propel it along the gut. Here, in the small intestine, the majority of nutrients are absorbed into the blood stream through the walls of the bowel. This is not smooth, but is covered with thousands of tiny *villi*, which are finger-like projections, and have the effect of greatly increasing the surface area of the bowel wall. The greater the surface area, the more nutrients can be absorbed.

Once the food residue enters the large intestine, fluid is

absorbed from the motions, and the residue of indigestible matter is propelled towards the rectum where it is stored until an appropriate time, and opportunity, for it to be passed out through the anus.

INFECTION (OTHERWISE KNOWN AS GASTRO-ENTERITIS)

That description of the bowel is, of course, what happens when everything is functioning normally, but with problems such as gastroenteritis everything changes dramatically. Gastroenteritis means that the lining of the digestive tract becomes irritated and inflamed.

Gastroenteritis is often also associated with vomiting. The child may have a raised temperature, and other members of the family or other contacts may also be suffering. Most gastroenteritis infections are caused by viruses, particularly a virus known as the rotavirus. However, they are sometimes caused by bacteria and other organisms. Diarrhoea can sometimes also result from eating toxic substances such as might be found in toadstools. Finally, even though hundreds of millions of bacteria are normally found in the healthy bowel, anything that changes this natural bacterial population of the bowel can also trigger off an episode of gastroenteritis. This could be, for instance, a course of some types of antibiotic.

Usually, but not always, the child with gastroenteritis is ill. He or she may have a fever, and possibly even blood or mucus in the motion. The only way anyone can tell for certain whether an infection is caused by a virus or bacteria is by examining a stool specimen. Incidentally, if your doctor suggests this, don't panic. He or she doesn't want a bucketful! You will be given a small specially designed specimen jar with a scoop.

Other infections occurring elsewhere in the body can also cause diarrhoea, especially in small children. Indeed, it can even be caused by such seemingly irrelevant problems as an ear infection.

DIETARY

Some children do seem particularly sensitive to particular foods or to a change in water. This seems to vary from family to family and child to child. Some children seem to develop tummy upsets if they go almost anywhere new, with the parents blaming it on curious causes such as 'a change in the water'. Other children never seem to get anything. When they were young, my wife and I took my children all over the world and I don't recall them ever getting any form of gastroenteritis.

Excessive drinking of fruit juices and sugary liquids might produce diarrhoea, as may weaning foods such as apple puree or mashed banana, which have high levels of fructose and are worth bearing in mind. Indeed there is a small but definite group of children, usually aged between six months and two years, who have persistent diarrhoea but are otherwise perfectly well. Paediatricians often call this the 'peas and carrots syndrome' – for fairly obvious reasons. Provided they are fit and otherwise healthy, and are growing normally, such children are not a cause for concern. Your doctor may ask to test the motions to exclude certain infections or conditions such as coeliac disease, but if these are normal they usually recover spontaneously.

When to consult a doctor

The single most important reason for seeking urgent medical attention for your child is dehydration.

The signs of dehydration are as follows:

- Very dry mouth
- Not passing urine for six hours or more
- Listless, apathetic, tired, sleepy
- Pale colour
- Sunken eyes

Dehydration is much more likely if the child is also vomiting as well as having diarrhoea. This is a medical emergency but is easily treated with fluid replacement. Despite this, children do still die of D&V in the U.K., and many millions of children die worldwide.

You should also always contact a doctor if your child has bloody diarrhoea. The most likely cause may be infection, but the doctor will want to exclude rarer causes such as intussusception – a type of bowel obstruction in babies.

If diarrhoea and vomiting continues for more than twenty-four hours without showing any sign of improving, then do at least contact your doctor for advice. You may be able to do this on the phone.

Gastroenteritis in adults and older children is a miserable inconvenience. In babies it can be fatal. In England and Wales it accounts for about ten per cent of all paediatric admissions to hospital. Most diarrhoea can be treated using the simple rehydration measures I describe in this chapter, but despite all the correct measures being used it can still persist for more than two or three days. Perhaps the most common cause for this is lactose intolerance. Lactose is the sugar in milk, and sometimes the virus causing the gastro-enteritis will temporarily destroy the intestine's ability to digest and absorb it. If it is not absorbed it can itself cause diarrhoea. In other words, although the original cause of the symptom has gone, the symptom continues.

If this is the case, stopping milk and all other lactose-containing products such as cheese and butter for a short while can bring about a speedy resolution of symptoms. Once the lactose is removed from the diet, both the diarrhoea and the intestine recover. Once the diarrhoea has stopped it is safe to reintroduce milk.

If diarrhoea goes on for more than four or five days, then your doctor might also ask you to collect a small sample of motion for analysis in the laboratory. Occasionally diarrhoea is caused by bacteria that can be helped by antibiotics. A bacteria known as campylobacter, which can easily be caught from pets, can cause diarrhoea and is easily cured by the antibiotic, erythromycin. However, as antibiotics will make many forms of diarrhoea worse, rather than better, doctors will want to know exactly which bacteria they are dealing with, rather than guessing. Hence the need for a specimen.

How you can help

The first line in treatment is to prevent the chief hazard, dehydration. So, give fluids. For a child who is drinking normally there should be no real problems. Children who are reluctant to drink or eat or who have profuse diarrhoea should be given special mixtures which contain dextrose and just the right amount of other salts and chemicals. These are marketed with trade names such as Dioralyte or Rehidrat, and are available on prescription, or can be purchased from chemist's shops. They consist of sachets of powder which should be mixed with the specified amounts of water. Despite what you may have heard, these really are dramatically better than simply giving water or ordinary squashes or soft drinks. Water, for instance, tends not to be very well absorbed if given by itself, because of the transport mechanism in the gut wall, and lemonade or cola drinks can actually make the diarrhoea worse, containing inadequate quantities of glucose and electrolytes to facilitate absorption.

If you cannot obtain these rehydration mixtures – if you are on holiday, for instance – Coca Cola diluted to half strength makes an acceptable substitute. As an approximate guide you should aim to give 150–200ml of fluid per kilogram of body weight per day. If kilograms still confuse you, a typical five-year-old boy weighs 18kg (40lb) and so should receive about three litres of fluid a day (approximately five pints).

A child with a fever requires even more fluid. For every two degrees Fahrenheit that his temperature goes up, his needs increase by ten per cent. Such fluid replacement has become the mainstay of the treatment of gastroenteritis, and simple as it seems it can be a lifesaver in infants. Antibiotics are generally worse than useless.

Do you starve or don't you? Doctors still seem totally divided. Some insist on nothing but boiled water or rehydration mixtures. Others say it simply doesn't matter. Certainly it has long been accepted that continued breast feeding is a good thing. Breast milk contains various chemicals, such as lymphocytes, interferon and other anti-infective factors, which may actually help speed recovery from the disease. Not only this, but it also contains calories and protein. Discontinuing breast feeding can also lead to the supply of breast milk actually drying up, so causing a long-term disadvantage for a short-term problem.

Apart from with very small children, I am a great believer that the body knows what it wants. If you get diarrhoea and don't feel hungry, don't eat. If you do, then it is almost certainly all right. Indeed, the majority of doctors now advise that children should be fed what they fancy – within reason! There is certainly no convincing evidence that starving either reduces the course of the disease or causes any other problems later on. Indeed, continuing to feed can help make the child feel better. It is bad enough feeling ill with a tummy upset. It is doubly bad if you feel hungry too!

Despite traditional advice, there is no need at all to reintroduce feeds gradually. No scientific studies have shown that this makes the least difference.

If your child has stomach pain with the diarrhoea, then paracetamol and a hot water bottle can be helpful, but if your child says his or her abdomen is tender when you touch it, you should seek medical advice.

Treatment

You will already have seen that by far the most important treatment is fluids. Most medication that has been used in the past to treat diarrhoea is either useless or potentially dangerous. I would go so far as to say that many treatments are about as much use as that recommended a hundred years ago by the President of the New York Medical Society. He suggested plugging the rectum with beeswax and oil cloth! Obviously this might appear to stop the diarrhoea, but has absolutely no effect on the cause, or on what is happening inside the abdomen.

Drugs such as kaolin are almost as useless, and more powerful drugs such as Lomotil may even be dangerous. They work by slowing the bowel down and stop the diarrhoea leaving the system. However they can have no effect on preventing the fluid accumulating in the intestine. Giving your child drugs like this may make you feel better – in that your child's diarrhoea may seem to stop – but is not really doing any good. Your child is still losing water and salts from his blood into the intestine, but you won't know about it and can feel falsely reassured. This type of drug can also stop the viruses or bacteria from being expelled from the bowel, and can have serious dangerous side effects, leading to severe muscular spasms.

Prevention

Hygiene is simply the most important preventative measure that you can take. Hygiene in the kitchen. Hygiene in the loo. In particular, teaching your children to wash hands after using the toilet. But occasional episodes of diarrhoea can never be entirely prevented.

PERSISTENT DIARRHOEA

Diarrhoea that goes on and on despite all the treatment and advice detailed here, will certainly need investigating. In infants this might be caused by coeliac disease, a condition where the child is unable to digest gluten-containing products (such as wheat or rye) and this obviously only starts when such foods have been given. Cystic fibrosis can also cause long-term diarrhoea in babies and will need investigating too.

In older children, diarrhoea that goes on a long time may well be the 'peas and carrots syndrome' that I described earlier, but your doctor may need to arrange referral or further investigations to rule out rarer conditions such as colitis.

The child with constipation

Symptoms

It is fair to say that the British have a thing about their bowels. It is almost as if they believe that there is some innate law that states that everyone shall go to the toilet every day without fail. In truth, this simply isn't the case at all. For adults, doctors consider that anything between having your bowels open three times a day and three times a week can be considered normal.

Nevertheless millions of pounds are spent every year on laxatives, and for most people they are so unnecessary that they might as well be flushed straight down the loo, so cutting out the middleman. Unfortunately, this obsessional anxiety about the possibility of constipation all too frequently gets passed on to our children.

Constipation simply means the infrequent passage of hard, dry, painful motions. If your child goes once every three days, is otherwise happy, is not in pain, and passes a normal but infrequent motion, then he or she is not ill, and is not constipated. And do not worry about any risk of toxins passing into the blood from retained motions. This is something of a myth. If your child seems happy, then please stop worrying. I'm really not terribly interested in how often your child goes to the loo, provided he or she is happy and well.

However, if passing a motion is painful, then you need to consider what the possible causes of this might be.

Causes

In any child, a brief spell of constipation is extremely common after almost any illness. This usually results from the child being off his or her food, as well as not drinking enough, and from sweating.

In infancy, breast feeding often causes infrequent motions, but the motions are usually loose. Bottle-fed babies, however, may develop constipation that is simply the result of their having a particular formula of milk, and it may be worth trying a switch of milk.

Persistent severe constipation starting from birth may be caused by lack of thyroid hormone, or from Hirschsprung's disease. In this relatively rare condition, which affects approximately one in every 5,000 babies, part of the bowel malfunctions because of a lack of nerve cells in a section of gut wall, and as a result the bowel does not contract normally. The condition may also be associated with abdominal swelling and vomiting.

In the second year of life apparent constipation is quite common, mainly because of the change in diet. However there can also be a problem with toilet training. Children may actually be frightened of passing a motion, and may try to avoid doing this. They may have a fear of the loo, embarrassment about going, and anxieties about what is actually happening when they pass a motion. In older children too, particularly when starting school, they may simply dislike cold unfamiliar loo seats, and crunchy loo paper – as one child described it to me.

Children with this problem of being frightened to pass a motion cannot hold back for ever. They may eventually pass a very large, very hard motion which can crack the skin of the anus (a condition known as an anal fissure). This can hurt a lot, making the child even more reluctant to pass motions again. A vicious circle can be set up. Going hurts, but not going leads to the build-up of an even bigger harder stool which is guaranteed to hurt even more. The child may go off his or her food, and there can even be soiling where loose motion seeps around the side of the harder blockage – often confusing parents into thinking that the child has diarrhoea, rather than constipation. This not uncommon situation results in a treatment that often puzzles parents – that of their child with apparent diarrhoea being treated with a laxative!

Other causes of constipation include not drinking enough, especially if the child has a fever. In addition, some children become constipated because their diet contains insufficient fibre. Unfortunately some parents, with all the best intentions, go too far with their insisting on their child taking fibre. Doctors refer to this rather disparagingly as the 'muesli belt syndrome'. A great deal of fibre, particularly using fibre supplements or high-fibre cereals, can actually be too much for young children. What they do need is fresh fruit, baked beans, wholemeal bread, and so on, not extra fibre supplements.

Some forms of medication can also cause constipation. Two examples are iron products used to treat anaemia (which can also make the motions black) and the so-called tri-cyclic drugs such as imipramine or amitryptyline which are sometimes used as part of the treatment of bedwetting.

When to consult a doctor

- The combination of constipation with vomiting may be a sign of obstruction, or blockage, of the bowel and should lead to you seeking medical advice right away.
- If you have a newborn baby who is persistently constipated with very hard stools.

- If a baby who is solely breast-fed is constipated.
- If your child passes blood in the motion. This should always be checked by a doctor, even though the most likely cause may well turn out to be an anal fissure, which is usually not serious.
- If you are concerned about your child's growth and development.
- If your child is unwell in any other way. In this case it is more likely that it is the unwellness that is causing the constipation, rather than the other way round.
- You might also seek medical advice if the constipation comes on after your child has been taking medication, or has had a change in diet – but this is often the sort of problem that can be dealt with on the telephone, or would be appropriate to discuss with your health visitor.

How you can help

In babies with constipation, one of the best treatments is pure fruit juice. Older children need enough fluid and enough fibre – green vegetables, baked beans, wholemeal bread, but not any form of fibre supplements. In addition, older children may well be helped by increasing their level of exercise – running and playing games, rather than sitting and playing Nintendo. After all, it is well known that there is no such thing as a constipated jogger.

Treatment

As in every condition, the doctor's treatment will depend on what is found at examination. The doctor will gently examine your child's abdomen, in particular feeling for fullness in the large intestine (the colon). The doctor may also need to perform a gentle rectal examination – feeling inside the anus using a lubricated, gloved little finger. Whilst obviously uncomfortable, this will only hurt if there is an anal fissure, and the doctor should be able to spot a fissure before inserting a finger.

The doctor may choose to prescribe a mild laxative, particularly a stool softener or lubricant if there is a fissure, or if passing a motion is painful. However I would advise you never to buy laxatives. These are almost always a complete waste of money, are usually completely unnecessary, and may indeed be harmful.

A very common problem is the one that actually results from the effectiveness of many laxatives. After taking the medicine, the child or adult passes a massive bowel motion. Following this the bowel is almost totally empty, and as a result the bowels do not need to be opened again for several days. The patient or parent therefore thinks that constipation is still a problem and takes yet more laxative. This can become a habit which goes on for fifty years or more. I know. I've got plenty of patients who've become stuck in this particularly unnecessary cycle of treatment.

Children with long-term constipation and associated soiling (known as encopresis) may well require hospital referral, long-term laxative drugs, and behavioural methods such as star charts to encourage a return to normal defecation. With a star chart, the child sticks a coloured star on a calendar every day that he or she does not soil, and is encouraged and praised for successful chart filling. Soiling is often dealt with in special hospital clinics run by both a doctor and a child psychologist. It can be a problem that takes many months to solve, but generally treatment is very effective.

Prevention

The key is diet. Fruit, vegetables, baked beans, fruit juice. Plenty of these and constipation is unlikely to be a problem. In addition, the other key to successful prevention is never to give your child any laxatives without seeking a doctor's advice. They cause far more problems than they ever solve.

The child with abnormal stools

Symptoms

Obviously, the two commonest types of abnormal stools are diarrhoea and constipation. Both of these problems have separate chapters devoted to them. In addition, in the section on diarrhoea I have included a brief introduction on how the bowels work which should help you understand the reasons that problems occur, and the rationale behind different treatments.

However there are other possible types of abnormal stools that this brief chapter will deal with. I will not subdivide this chapter in the usual way, but will deal with each type of abnormal stool in full – one at a time.

The main possible problems are:

- Blood in the stools
- Abnormal coloured stools
- Threadworms
- Abnormally textured stools
- Fatty stools

BLOOD IN THE STOOLS

In reality bleeding can either be in the stool or on the stool, a subtle difference which can be vitally important in unravelling the cause.

Causes

By far the commonest cause of blood on the stool is an anal

fissure. This is a tiny crack in the anus, usually caused by constipation. As the motion comes through the anus it stretches the crack open still further, and this leads to a small bleed. This may be on the motion, or may just be seen on the nappy or pants. Such bleeding causes parents tremendous anxiety, but is rarely important and usually gets better rapidly.

There may be slightly more bleeding from a polyp (a small growth from the lining of the bowel that may project on a stalk) in the intestine, or from a condition known as a Meckel's diverticulum. This condition is present in about one child in every fifty, but typically causes no symptoms at all. Before the baby is born, there is a connection between the umbilical cord and the intestine through the navel. The intestinal end of this tube can persist after birth, as a small blind sac attached to the small intestine. Whilst it is usually harmless, occasionally it can lead to bleeding, or conditions such as intussusception or volvulus. (Volvulus is described in the section on abdominal pain.)

Intussusception is a condition that typically occurs between the ages of three months and nine months. In it, part of the bowel telescopes inside itself. Imagine an opened telescope being slowly closed. Now imagine doing that with a length of bowel. The bowel reacts by creating increasing muscular spasm, as if it were trying to move the swelling along and out, but, of course, this simply has the effect of making the problem get worse and worse. The symptoms of intussusception are therefore severe colicky abdominal pain, associated with the passage of very bloody motions. For some curious reason, doctors often describe pathological conditions by comparing them to foodstuffs. The stool of intussusception is described as a redcurrant jelly stool. Revolting, but accurate! Intussusception can follow an episode of gastroenteritis, or an upper respiratory infection which has caused enlarged glands in the abdomen.

When to consult a doctor

You should always consult a doctor if your child passes any blood, or there is blood on the motion. However the passage of a large amount of blood, or a 'redcurrant jelly stool' is a medical emergency and you should seek medical help immediately.

Treatment

Treatment will depend on the exact cause, but if the cause of bleeding is an anal fissure, the most important solution is to keep the child's motions loose. Your doctor may prescribe a mild laxative, if diet is not enough, and also an anaesthetic cream to numb any pain from the fissure. Stopping the pain is important or constipation is likely to follow.

ABNORMAL COLOURED STOOLS

New parents are often astonished by the extraordinary technicolor stools that their babies pass. In the first weeks stools can vary from bright green or bright yellow, both of which are normal.

White

White stools in a child who looks sun-tanned may be a sign of jaundice, particularly if the child is also passing darker urine than normal.

Green

Green stools in older children are usually harmless as long as they only happen occasionally. They often occur in children with diarrhoea and are just a sign that the bowel motions have passed so quickly through the gut that the bile has not had time to be chemically changed into the brown colour of normal motions. If green motions occur repeatedly, then do seek medical advice.

Red

When children pass red stools, parents usually assume that this is caused by blood (see beginning of this chapter), but in fact there may be other causes. The commonest are red foodstuffs, in particular beetroot and red liquorice, and in children with diarrhoea the redness of tomato soup or red jellies may show through. In addition a number of medicines and vitamins may colour the motions red.

Black

Medication can also be the cause of black stools – iron products are a common culprit. Black motions may also result from liquorice, or spinach, and children who make a habit of eating coal may – hardly surprisingly – pass black motions. (Incidentally, eating dirt, coal, and similar substances may be a sign of anaemia, so do report this to your doctor.)

The most important cause of black motions is bleeding into the bowel. Bleeding into the first part of the bowel, in particular the stomach or small intestine, does not appear at the anus as red blood. Instead, it is affected by the bowel contents and acid, becoming black and tarry. You should always contact a doctor if a child who looks or feels unwell passes black motions, especially if the child also complains of abdominal pain.

THREADWORMS

You may notice threadworms on your child's motions. Threadworms are so named because they look like tiny pieces of cotton thread, and the first reaction of almost every patient on spotting these is one of horror and embarrassment. Well, don't be horrified. Don't be embarrassed. Threadworms are incredibly common. Almost every family will have suffered from these at some time, and they are neither harmful nor a sign of any form of negligence on your part.

Incidentally, not all white thread-like matter in the faeces is necessarily a threadworm. Bananas can cause a similar appearance. If in doubt, ask your doctor. The worms – or banana threads – can be captured by sticking a piece of sticky tape against the anus in the morning shortly after waking, then transferring the tape to a slide for examination under a microscope.

The following section does not make for pleasant reading, but understanding the life cycle of threadworms is important to understanding how they should be eradicated. Threadworms live in the bowel, and at night the females emerge through the anus to lay their eggs on the skin around the anus. (How they know that it is night is one of life's unsolved mysteries.) This leads to itching, scratching, and frequently to disturbed sleep.

The child will almost certainly then get the threadworm eggs on his or her finger, and then put the fingers in the mouth so swallowing more eggs and worsening the problem. The problem is also extremely infectious around families, as the eggs can become part of the household dust and are therefore easily transferred from one family member to another. For this reason, doctors will always treat the whole family to stop re-infection.

The chief symptom of threadworms is anal itching. In girls the threadworms can also affect the urethra and vagina causing itching there. Threadworms do not cause illness, or weight loss. Many people have fantasies of the worms living in the bowel eating the food that the sufferer takes in. This is absolute nonsense.

Treatment

Treatment consists of medication such as Pripsen (piperazine) or Vermox (mebendazole). This is taken as a single dose, and usually repeated a couple of weeks later. You should check with your doctor if you are pregnant, or any of the children needing treatment are aged under one. It is also important that bedding and pyjamas are washed at the same time to clear away any remaining eggs, and scrupulous hygiene, trimming of fingernails, and ensuring the whole family is treated will all ensure rapid recovery.

ABNORMALLY TEXTURED STOOLS

At the time that a child starts to eat solids, all sorts of remarkable changes can occur in the appearance of the texture of the motions. Fruits, particularly pears, can cause a curious gritty appearance which is completely harmless. If older children develop gritty-looking motions this may well be a sign of pica, or dirt eating – and this in itself may be a sign of iron-deficiency anaemia. You certainly should consult a doctor if you are in doubt about the cause of your child's unusual stools.

FATTY STOOLS

Children may occasionally pass motions that are so fatty and greasy that they are almost impossible to flush away. This condition, known as steatorrhoea, is caused by a failure of the body to absorb fat from the diet, a problem known as malabsorption. This has a number of other consequences, including weight loss, poor appetite, slow development or anaemia. By far the commonest cause of malabsorption is coeliac disease, and this typically becomes obvious in the first two years of life – though it may not become obvious until much later. I once had a woman patient in whom it was diagnosed at the age of seventy-two and who had probably suffered from it all her life!

Coeliac disease is caused by a sensitivity to gluten, the germ protein in wheat. The lining of the bowel appears to be damaged through this sensitivity, and it shrinks. The finger-like villi which normally greatly increase the surface area of the bowel lining disappear and because there is so much less area for absorption, many nutrients fail to be absorbed. Once the diagnosis has been proven by a doctor, the treatment is a gluten-free diet.

The child with abdominal pain

Symptoms

Abdominal pain in children can either be a one-off episode of pain (known as 'acute' pain) or alternatively it may be recurrent (known as 'chronic' pain). This chapter will deal with these separately.

ONE-OFF ABDOMINAL PAIN

Causes

All children get abdominal pain at times. 'Tummy ache' must be one of the most common complaints, and it usually fades away harmlessly. Abdominal pain also frequently is associated with diarrhoea and sickness – and these topics are dealt with in separate chapters. Tummy ache caused by 'something he ate' usually disappears after a few hours. Whilst sudden abdominal pain can certainly be frightening both for the child and his or her parents, the cause is often simple and harmless, like an attack of wind.

However, pain that steadily gets worse and worse over a matter of hours may well be more significant. There are any number of possible causes – from appendicitis (see page 150) to constipation. I am not even going to attempt to teach you how to diagnose abdominal pain as, even after many years' experience, doctors still can find it extremely difficult to distinguish between appendicitis and other less important conditions. However, what you do need to know is when you should call a doctor. Following this I will give details of a few of the more important common conditions which should be of some help after the doctor has made the diagnosis.

When to call a doctor

- If pain is severe and doesn't ease up
- If pain is constant for more than a couple of hours
- If pain that has been crampy becomes constant
- If a child continues to retch even after there is nothing left to bring up
- If your child seems to be very ill
- If it hurts when you press on your child's abdomen
- If your child's abdomen is swollen
- If there is a history of any injury to the abdomen
- If your child's abdomen feels rock hard
- If a boy has any pain in the testicles
- If there is any blood in your child's motions or vomit

RECURRENT ABDOMINAL PAIN

Causes

The commonest cause of recurrent abdominal pain is a curious condition known as the 'periodic syndrome'. The cause is far from certain, but the condition affects up to fifteen per cent of school-aged children. The pain is typically worse in the day, and doesn't disturb sleep. It can continue on and off for months.

The most likely explanation is that some children are either more sensitive to the normal contractions of the gut ('peristalsis') or have stronger than average contractions. It is not caused by constipation, though constipation can sometimes result from it.

A number of other conditions tend to occur in a family, and these include migraine, ulcers, and colitis. Stress can worsen the pain, though it is unlikely that it is the sole cause. In some children, tummy ache can be the equivalent of an adult's headache. Sometimes the pain is worsened by particular foods, such as wheat, milk products, or some artificial sweeteners – though food intolerance is also likely to cause symptoms such as bloating and diarrhoea. I cover these in detail elsewhere in the book. If you think that constipation is the problem, then do see the separate section in this book on that condition (on page 134).

When to consult a doctor

All children with recurrent abdominal pain should be assessed by a doctor, even though frequently all the tests are negative. In particular, every child with recurrent abdominal pain should have his or her urine examined to make sure there is no sign of infection.

The child with the periodic syndrome rarely has any other symptoms, such as diarrhoea, vomiting, weight loss, fever, or anything else. If these occur, then do consult your doctor, and remember that having the periodic syndrome doesn't give your child exemption from other abdominal problems. He or she could still get appendicitis, for instance, so if the symptoms change, seek help.

In summary, consult your doctor if your child has chronic pain, but consult again if any of the following occur:

- The pain changes – either in timing, severity, or position
- There is vomiting
- Your child wakes at night in pain
- Your child also complains of joint pains or aching
- Your child's abdomen appears to be swollen
- The stools are black or tarry

- Your child doesn't seem to be growing as fast as normal (either weight or height)

SPECIFIC CAUSES OF ABDOMINAL PAIN

This section only deals with five of the more common causes of pain. Unfortunately, there is an almost limitless list of possible causes of abdominal pain and if I don't discuss your child's problem here then do ask your doctor if she or he can provide more information. The topics considered here are:

- Appendicitis
- Colic
- Intussusception
- Mesenteric adenitis
- Intussusception and volvulus

Appendicitis

The appendix is a blind tube, about three to four inches long, which is situated at the beginning of the large intestine at the bottom right-hand corner of the abdomen. Inflammation of the appendix must be one of the best known surgical conditions, though the appendix itself is now somewhat redundant as it no longer has any significant function in humans.

Typically the symptoms start with a vague central tummy ache, with the pain being located around the area of the umbilicus. The child may then be sick, and the pain will shift to the bottom right of the abdomen, where it gradually increases in intensity. Most children with appendicitis will have a slight fever. In addition, your child is likely to refuse food and drink, and the breath may well be foul-smelling.

All of that sounds very straightforward, and you would

think that diagnosis should be easy, but whilst appendicitis can be the easiest condition for a doctor to diagnose, it can also be the hardest. If your child has symptoms that could be appendicitis, then your G.P. may well choose to admit him or her to hospital. However, unless it is absolutely clear that this is the diagnosis, your child may initially simply be observed. A significant proportion of episodes of pain that sound exactly like appendicitis just seem to fade away. (Though never assume that this will happen without involving a doctor.) Even when surgery is restricted to the most clear-cut and definite cases and the appendix is removed, quite a large proportion will turn out to have a normal appendix. On the other side of the story, a significant number of episodes of abdominal pain that don't sound in the very least like appendicitis turn out to be this condition! Indeed, there isn't a doctor in the world who hasn't been fooled by appendicitis! When the diagnosis of appendicitis is confirmed, there is only one treatment, and that is surgery.

Colic

Symptoms

Sometimes known as 'three-month-colic' as it occurs primarily in the first twelve weeks of life, colic involves repeated episodes of crying and even screaming in a baby who is otherwise perfectly well. In a typical episode the baby is tense and rigid as he or she cries. Frequently the child will scream, and parents often say that they recognise this as an entirely different cry to normal. In addition, your baby may pull his or her knees up, and the pain will seem to come in paroxysms, with lots of wind being passed after an attack.

No one is really sure what the cause of colic is. Some doctors even seem to doubt its existence, though as a parent who has had to tolerate the screaming of two colicky babies, I am not one of them! It is quite likely that it is not so much a disease as a symptom with lots of different possible causes. There is now some thought that it may just be a phase of development that babies go through, rather than an illness. The great majority of babies with colic are happy and healthy and well in every other way. In particular, it is fair to say that if they are gaining weight and thriving there is unlikely to be anything significant wrong.

Causes

Entire books have been written about the possible causes of colic, and ways of treating it. Most parents believe that the underlying problem is something to do with 'wind'. This certainly seems logical. After all, they seem bloated and often pass wind at the end of a bout of screaming. However it may not be as simple as this. It is clear that crying in itself makes some babies gulp air down between episodes of screaming, and it is possible that the wind may be a result of all the crying rather than the cause. There is certainly no real evidence that colicky babies have more wind than any other babies.

When to consult a doctor

I believe that all colicky babies should be checked over by a doctor at least once. The doctor may find nothing wrong, nor have much new in the way of treatment, but it is important to make sure that the diagnosis is correct. In addition, if colic seems to go on in a child over four months of age then the diagnosis may not be colic and you should seek advice.

Treatment

So, if no one is certain about the cause, how can you help it? Many children experience considerable relief from colic drops such as Infacol, which can be very effective. Some herbal treatments – such as fennel – may help, but do seek advice before using these. Your health visitor will probably be able to help. In addition, there is some suggestion that cows' milk products can aggravate colic, so it is worth a trial of avoiding this if the colic is severe. Talk to your doctor or health visitor before trying soya-based milks as a substitute for your normal baby milk. If you are breast feeding, you could try avoiding dairy products yourself. This can make a very real difference.

Intussusception

In intussusception, a condition which can occur at any age but which is commonest between three and nine months, one part of the intestine slides inside the part next to it, just like a telescope being collapsed. The bowel contracts to try and move this swelling along, and as a result even more bowel becomes intussuscepted.

Symptoms

The symptoms are typical. The child has severe, colicky, abdominal pain often followed by vomiting and the passing of stools that look just like redcurrant jelly.

The problem typically follows a viral infection, and always has to be managed in hospital. The child may initially be given a barium enema – a type of X-ray that can confirm the diagnosis, and which can sometimes be enough to straighten the bowel out, though surgery is needed very frequently.

Intussusception is not common, but it is serious, relatively easy to diagnose, and once it has been treated it leaves no significant after effects.

Mesenteric adenitis

Although you may not have heard the term 'mesenteric adenitis', it is actually very common. This is the type of abdominal pain that typically occurs in children when they have a throat infection. Everyone is aware that when you get a throat infection, the lymph glands in the neck swell up to prevent the infection spreading elsewhere. These infection-fighting glands are also present along the intestine, and during any infection – even an infection elsewhere in the body, such as in the throat – these too can swell up. Sometimes the pain that they cause can be every bit as severe as the pain of appendicitis. Typically this fades after thirty-six to forty-eight hours, and leaves no after effects.

Volvulus

Volvulus is the term used to describe the twisting of part of the bowel on itself. In the same way that twisting a hosepipe would stop water flowing through it, volvulus leads to an obstruction of the bowel, leading to vomiting and severe abdominal pain, and occasionally bleeding in the motion. Volvulus needs hospital assessment, and usually requires an operation. The condition can be serious, because – as well as blocking the passage of the gut contents – the twisting can also cut off the blood supply to that section of the gut, causing gangrene.

The child with problems passing urine

Symptoms

This chapter will deal with a number of related symptoms. These are:

- Pain passing urine
- Frequent passing of urine
- Offensive smelling urine
- Discoloured urine – including blood in the urine
- Bedwetting
- Dribbling urine

As one of the most important causes of many of these symptoms is a urinary tract infection, I shall devote a separate section to these infections.

However, before going into these problems in detail, it is worth briefly summarising the anatomy of the urinary system. Urine is formed in the kidneys, which are to be found in the back just underneath the rib cage. The urine then passes down two tubes – called the ureters – into the bladder. The bladder is a muscular bag and it is found in the centre of the very lowest part of the abdomen. Urine slowly collects in the bladder, and when it is full, messages are sent by the nervous system to the brain and the sensation of 'needing to go to the toilet' is felt. (Incidentally, these nerves are really only able to transmit one sensation, so irritation or infection of the walls of the bladder creates exactly the same sensation as happens when the bladder is full and makes the sufferer feel that he or she needs to pass urine, even if there is little or no urine present.) Finally, the urine is passed from the bladder into the urethra, which is the tube that leads to the outside – either in the upper vulval area or at the end of the penis. The urethra is obviously longer in males than in females, as it has to stretch the length of the penis, and for reasons that I will explain this is the reason why females get more urine infections than males. This difference in length of the urethra is obviously more significant in men than it is in toddlers.

PAIN PASSING URINE

Causes

If your child complains of pain on passing urine, by far the most likely cause is an infection in the urine. Whilst I will deal with urine infections in some detail shortly, I must stress that it is absolutely essential that this diagnosis is not guessed at, but is properly assessed and investigated by a doctor. If a child has symptoms that you decide are likely to be caused by a urine infection, whatever you do, do not just give him or her some antibiotics that you might have left over from some other infection, or from another child. This could be genuinely harmful for your child.

When to consult a doctor

Every child who complains of pain on passing urine should therefore have a specimen of urine examined by the doctor to exclude infection.

How you can help

There are other conditions which can cause pain. Irritation

of the urethra can cause pain, and this irritation could result from, for instance, chemicals in the bath water inflaming the lower urethra in girls. Such chemicals could include shampoos and bubble bath, and if your child is prone to this then restrict the use of bubble baths, try to avoid soap coming into contact with the vulval area, wash hair at the end, rather than the beginning, of bath time, and if possible encourage your child to pass urine after getting out of the bath as this will flush the urethra clear.

Other things that can irritate the urethra include bicycle seats, sand, and over-vigorous wiping after using the toilet, especially in girls who wipe themselves from the back towards the front rather than the other way round.

FREQUENT PASSING OF URINE

As children get older, they gradually pass urine less frequently. Whilst infants pass urine up to twenty times in twenty-four hours, two-year-olds will only go about ten times in the same period, and by the teenage years most people are only going about five times a day.

Causes

A number of conditions can make children pass urine more frequently. These are:

Increased fluid intake

The child who drinks more fluid than normal, possibly because of habit or suddenly developing a passion for a particular drink, is bound to pass more urine.

Drugs and other chemicals

Caffeine (in cola drinks, coffee or tea) stimulates more frequent urination. Some treatments used in asthma or hay-fever can also have a similar effect.

Diabetes

An unexplained onset of excessive thirst and frequent passing of urine are important signs of diabetes. However, children who develop diabetes are usually generally unwell, losing weight and frequently being excessively hungry.

Anxiety or stress

Think back to when you took an exam at school, or even took your driving test or had some other stressful occasion. You almost certainly felt the need to keep going to the toilet beforehand, even though when you got there there was little or no urine to pass. Stress has a powerful effect on the need to pass urine, which is all part of the body's 'fight or flight' response to stress. Faced with a problem, our bodies are conditioned either to run away, or to stand and fight, and so the heart races, the bladder is emptied, breathing speeds up, and so on. All these are entirely inappropriate for the average stress that we face in the late twentieth century, but our bodies have not yet fully adapted to modern forms of stress.

If your child is feeling particularly stressed for any reason – problems at school, problems at home, a new baby in the family, excitement before a holiday, or almost anything else – then he or she may well pass urine more frequently. However it is unlikely for this to interfere with sleep, whereas other causes of frequency, such as infection, may well cause frequent urination during the night as well as in the day.

A very unusual cause of a child frequently passing urine is if he or she has developed an obsession with hand-washing, and is actually going to the toilet or bathroom to wash the hands rather than actually passing urine.

Urine infection

This is a common and important cause of frequent urination and is dealt with in detail at the end of this chapter.

OFFENSIVE SMELLING URINE

Causes

This may well be a sign of a urine infection, particularly if the smell is fishy or otherwise unpleasant. However there are other causes of smelly urine and these include:

Foods – such as asparagus

Drugs – particularly antibiotics

Stale urine in nappies

Metabolic disorders – some very rare congenital problems which result in abnormal metabolism can cause curious smelling urine right from early infancy

When to consult a doctor

If your child has abnormal smelling urine, have a look at the section in this chapter on urine infections. If he or she has any other symptoms, then collect a specimen of your child's urine and consult your doctor.

DISCOLOURED URINE – INCLUDING BLOOD IN THE URINE

Causes

Your child may pass urine in an assortment of colours, and each of these colours has a different significance.

Deep yellow

Darker coloured urine is normally a sign of the urine being more concentrated. This can happen because your child has not been drinking enough fluids, or if he or she is sweating excessively. The child with a fever – whatever the cause – is likely to sweat more, and if this is not compensated for by drinking plenty of fluid, then the urine will look very dark.

Persistent very dark urine, that can look the colour of very strong tea, may be a sign of liver problems such as hepatitis. In these conditions the child is also likely to look jaundiced.

Red

The most important cause of red urine is blood in the urine. This may be a sign of a urine infection, but may also be caused by kidney stones, or trauma to the kidneys.

However all that is red is not blood! Many parents get very frightened when their child passes bright red urine, and are then relieved when they discover that the cause is simply the fact that the child has been eating beetroot! A number of food colourings can cause red urine, as may eating a lot of blackberries, some antibiotics, and some fruit drinks.

Occasionally children may pass a dark, mahogany-coloured urine, if they have had significant damage to muscle. This can occur after trauma, after the severe muscle spasm that occurs in an epileptic fit, or various other problems. Your child should be assessed by a doctor. Please take a urine specimen with you when you attend.

Your doctor can perform a simple test on the urine to determine whether the red colour is caused by blood or not. The doctor will use a very sensitive testing stick, or arrange for the urine to be examined under a microscope to determine if there are blood cells present.

Black

The urine may appear to be black in some children who eat rhubarb, who take some forms of medication, and in an unusual type of metabolic problem that is present from birth. In alcaptonuria the urine turns black after it is left to stand, or if it is left in a nappy for a while. This can produce the puzzling situation where a baby may be found to have black colouring in the nappies, but if the parent sees the baby pass urine it looks completely normal as it comes out.

Blue

Blue urine usually results from food colourings, particularly when large amounts of highly coloured food is eaten. The most typical scenario is after a birthday party when huge quantities of brightly coloured birthday cake is consumed.

Green

This too can be linked with the more lurid food colourings.

Pink

Pink urine can be caused by some types of medication (particularly laxatives that contain phenolphthalein), as well as beetroot and blackberries.

Cloudy urine

If you collect a sample of your child's urine and store it in the refrigerator before taking it to your doctor, you may well notice some crystals appear. These are entirely harmless, and will usually disappear if the urine is warmed back up to room temperature. In addition, urine also may well appear to be cloudy if your child has not been drinking much fluid.

Cloudiness in urine at room temperature, on the other hand, is likely to be caused by a urine infection, and so you should consult your doctor. Infection is not inevitable, however, as some children do seem to excrete more chemicals into their urine and have cloudy but otherwise normal urine. If the child drinks more fluid, this cloudiness is likely to disappear.

Incidentally, the appearance of crystals in the urine in a nappy is a problem that a number of worried parents have consulted me about. This is almost always caused by some of the absorbent gel that can be part of the modern super-absorbent nappies, and which can occasionally pass through the nappy itself, especially if it is slightly torn.

BEDWETTING

Bedwetting can cause enormous anxiety for both parents and children. Otherwise known as nocturnal enuresis, it can turn bedtime from being the relaxed enjoyable time that we would like it to be into a stressful time of anxiety and argument. The child whose every trip to bed ends in his feeling embarrassed and upset is hardly likely to look forward to bedtime with eager anticipation.

Bedwetting only becomes a problem when a child continues to wet at night after the majority have become dry. There is no sudden dividing line between the normal and abnormal. And whilst I can describe the natural history of acquiring bladder control, remember that this only describes the 'average' child. The child who does not fit this schedule exactly is not necessarily abnormal.

The very young infant has virtually no bladder control. The bladder gradually fills, and when it is sufficiently distended it empties. Indeed it is rare for the child to have any significant bladder control before he or she can walk. After all, if you can't get to the pot, there is no point in waiting. Around fifteen to eighteen months the child usually becomes able to tell his or her mother that he or she has wet his nappy, and shortly afterwards says he or she wants to go, but doesn't give her time to do anything about it. By eighteen to twenty-four months he or she is able to tell his or her mother in time to be got to the pot or lavatory, and by two to two and a half he or she can go alone. The three-year-old may be able to get through the night dry if he is potted at his parents' bedtime.

Approximately nine out of ten children become dry at night sometime between one and a half and four years, usually sometime during the third year. Control of bowel function comes before control of the bladder, and even after becoming dry all children can temporarily become wet if they are stressed.

Bedwetting tends to cause numerous problems for parents. After all the child who is deeply asleep tends to empty his or her bladder completely, leaving a bed that is not merely damp but soaking. The problems of laundry, of smells, and of the general management of the mess can make a mother despair – particularly if she is simply told by doctors or friends that her child will grow out of it.

Causes

There are numerous different theories as to why bedwetting occurs. These vary from the psychological to the physical, and when there are so many explanations for something you can be pretty sure none of them is totally correct. However, some things are clear. There is certainly no evidence that children who wet their bed are neurotic. Physical causes are also unusual, particularly in the child who only wets at night. Children who have daytime problems with passing urine as well as night-time problems do need closer assessment. The most likely explanation is delayed maturation. Some children are simply dryer later than others. In exactly the same way that some children walk later than others. Delayed maturation probably is also affected by social factors, emotional factors, and, rarely, physical causes.

When to consult a doctor

If your child gets to the age of five years and is still wetting at night then you should consult a doctor. In addition, you should consult if a child who has previously been dry suddenly becomes wet, or if the child complains of any pain on passing urine, or if it is causing very real upset for either of you.

The doctor will almost certainly initially test a urine specimen to make sure there is no infection. Following this, there are a large number of possible treatments. These include star charts, medication, and buzzer alarms. The buzzer can be particularly effective, and consists of a sensor pad that goes in the bed and detects the presence of urine or moisture. This sets an alarm off which wakes the child up. After a few nights, the child wakes before the alarm goes off – although frequently the rest of the house wakes up as well. None of the treatments is guaranteed as being effective, but most are worth trying.

Many children are not terribly worried about bedwetting, but are concerned if they are going to stay with friends or are going on a trip from school. On these occasions your doctor may be able to prescribe medication that interferes with the production of urine overnight. This includes Desmospray nasal spray, and DDAVP tablets. These have no long-term effect, but may give the child confidence and avoid tremendous embarrassment.

How you can help

Before a child is five years old there is really very little point in trying any particular therapies to make them dry at night. Think about it. If the cause is delayed maturation, then no amount of encouragement will make the child mature quicker. If a child is late walking, however much you might encourage him or her to walk, he or she will only walk when the time is right – and the same probably applies to dryness at night. It has been calculated that fifty per cent of three-year-olds, ten per cent of six-year-olds, and only three per cent of ten-year-olds will be wet during the night.

If your child is occasionally dry at night, then he or she may nearly be ready to become totally dry. You might want to try 'star charts'. This is a simple diary chart, and every time the child is dry at night he or she puts a coloured star on the appropriate night. The system I use gives a blue star for every dry night, and a red star if there are three dry nights in a row. This can be extraordinarily effective, but only if the child is ready.

Bedwetting is certainly frustrating and upsetting, but in general the less fuss you make the better. At least this will lower the emotional temperature. Incidentally, I have never been convinced that cutting out night-time drinks makes the least difference. If anything, this makes the problem worse. The child goes to bed thirsty, dehydrated, and with the whole problem of bedwetting at the forefront of their mind. Treat them normally. In addition, as is detailed elsewhere in this chapter, restricted fluid intake can predispose to urine infections – something that will guarantee to make bedwetting even worse.

DRIBBLING URINE

If your child – whatever the age – always seems to be dribbling small amounts of urine, then you should very definitely consult a doctor. Whilst occasional wetting is obviously not at all unusual, constant dribbling may be a sign either of some form of abnormality in the bladder or urethra, or possibly of the nervous supply to the bladder. It needs investigation.

URINARY TRACT INFECTIONS

In several sections of this chapter I have mentioned the importance of urinary tract infection. This section will deal with this in some detail.

Symptoms

The main symptoms of a urinary tract infection (typically

abbreviated to U.T.I., and which refers to infection in the urine, bladder, urethra, ureter, and/or kidneys) may be any of the following:

- Frequency (passing urine more frequently than normal)
- Pain on passing urine
- Offensive smelling urine
- Blood in the urine
- Back pain
- Tummy ache – which can be very vague and nondescript. For this reason, every child with an undiagnosed tummy ache should have their urine tested
- Fever
- Bedwetting
- In addition, babies may just be vaguely unwell, possibly off their food, and may also have vomiting or diarrhoea

Causes

Bacteria almost always get into the bladder from the outside, up the urethra. The bacteria concerned are typically germs from the bowel, and when you consider the short distance between the anus and the urethra, it is somewhat surprising that infections do not happen even more frequently. Because the urethra is so much shorter in girls than boys, bacteria are more likely to be able to pass up into the bladder. Indeed, approximately one out of twenty girls will have a U.T.I. before they reach puberty.

If the infection only affects the bladder, this is termed cystitis ('cyst' meaning bladder, '–itis' meaning inflammation). If the infection gets up the ureters to one or both kidneys, then this infection is termed pyelonephritis.

When to consult a doctor

Every small child who might have a urinary infection should be seen by a doctor. There should be no exceptions to this rule. First of all, the diagnosis is not always easy to make just from the symptoms. The urine has to be examined to confirm the presence or absence of infection. If there is a proven infection, then almost every child will then be investigated to make sure there is no abnormality of the urinary tract, such as an ineffective valve at the bottom of the ureter. It is vitally important to know that there is no risk of recurrent infections, or of any long-term damage to the kidneys. The fact that most children do not have any significant problems is neither here nor there. Finding, and treating, children who might be at long-term risk of kidney damage is enormously worthwhile.

Whilst you should always consult a doctor if there is any possibility of urine infection, you should see a doctor *urgently* if your child's temperature is over 38.3°C, if he or she is complaining of abdominal pain, if there is blood in the urine, or if your child seems ill.

The doctor may initially test the urine using testing sticks, which can detect the presence of blood, nitrites (which are present if bacteria are in the urine), glucose, and protein. Some tests also look for the presence of white blood cells, which indicate pus. The specimen is also likely to be sent to the local laboratory, where it will be examined under a microscope, and any bacteria will be cultured to determine what antibiotics they might be sensitive to.

If infection is definitely confirmed, then children aged under five will always have this investigated further, typically using an ultrasound scan to look at the kidneys, ureters, and bladder (known as a K.U.B. scan). This scan is designed to look for problems like ureteric reflux. There are normally valves that allow urine to pass down ureters into bladder, but not back up ureters from bladder. In some children these valves may not be working properly, and infected urine can flow up into the ureters and so infect the kidneys. This reflux may predispose the kidneys to recurrent infection, scarring, and permanent long-term damage. This is not common, but always detectable. Incidentally, infections that occur after the age of six years are very unlikely indeed to lead to kidney damage, and so investigation is much less important.

How you can help

If you suspect a urine infection, as well as consulting a doctor you should also strongly encourage your child to drink as much as he or she possibly can. This helps to flush the kidneys and bladder out. Collect a fresh urine specimen in a sterile bottle just before you go to the doctor's, though this is obviously tricky in small babies and the doctor may be able to provide you with special stick-on bags that make the task very much more easy.

Treatment

As well as extra fluids, antibiotics are absolutely essential for the treatment of proven infections. Even if normally you try to avoid antibiotics for your child, and use homoeopathic or herbal remedies, I would ask you to allow antibiotics to be used for this particular condition. The potential for long-term kidney damage in untreated urine infection is very real, and can cause your child major problems for the rest of his or her life. Sometimes infections are recurrent, and if this occurs your child may need repeated courses of antibiotics or even a prolonged course of treatment at a low dose.

Prevention

Children who are prone to urine infection should increase their day-to-day fluid intake. In addition, girls should be encouraged to wipe themselves from front to back when they go to the toilet. Wiping from back to front can transfer bacteria from the anus to the opening of the urethra, whereas wiping front to back carries no such risk.

The child with problems with the genitals or groin

This chapter will deal with the following problems:

Boys
- The absent or disappearing testicle
- Problems with the foreskin
- Problems with the scrotum
- Problems with the penis
- Injuries to the genitals

Girls
- Vaginal itching
- Vaginal bleeding
- Vaginal discharge
- Foreign bodies in the vagina
- Problems with the labia
- Injuries to the genitals

Both boys and girls
- Swellings in the groin

PROBLEMS WITH BOYS' GENITALS

The absent or disappearing testicle

One testicle always hangs slightly lower than the other, and this is entirely normal. If you notice that one, or even both, of the testicles never appears to be in the scrotum, then do consult a doctor. If left for many years, an undescended testicle may be permanently damaged.

However, many boys have testicles that appear and disappear from the scrotum like a yo-yo going up and down. This is because the testicles are attached to sensitive muscles, which pull the testicles up out of harm's way – particularly if they are exposed to cold, or if the child is embarrassed at being exposed. Many boys appear to have missing testicles when assessed at school medicals, but this is frequently because a doctor who is a stranger examines them with cold hands – a perfect recipe for disappearance.

If you want to check whether your child's testicles are in the scrotum, then a warm bath is the ideal opportunity. If a testicle can ever be found in the scrotum, then there is rarely any cause for concern. If it *can* be there, it will be there when it matters.

Problems with the foreskin

Many problems with the foreskin result from well-meaning but faulty advice. Do not try to forcefully pull back your child's foreskin so that you can clean under it. You should only pull it back – very gently – as far as it will naturally go. If you pull it further there is a risk of scarring developing which will cause problems later on. Incidentally, it is not uncommon for the foreskin not to retract completely until the age of ten years.

If the foreskin has been pulled back forcefully there is a very real risk of it becoming stuck behind the head of the penis, where it swells up. This condition is known as paraphimosis. As the foreskin swells, it squeezes harder on the penis, which swells up even further, and a very painful vicious circle gets set up. This is a condition that requires urgent medical attention.

Sometimes the foreskin will swell up in its normal position. This can be caused by trapping the foreskin in a zip (ouch!), or by poor hygiene, or soap being left under the foreskin after washing. If there is pus oozing out, or if the foreskin is hot or tender, then seek medical help. If it is painless and not particularly red, then gentle washing with warm water can help. Let him soak in a bath, though do *not* add bubble bath or use soap.

Many boys who have not been circumcised produce a white cheesy material that forms naturally under the edge of the foreskin. This is entirely harmless, and nothing to be concerned about.

Some boys do have a foreskin that is too tight, although only relatively few need to have a circumcision. The main sign that the foreskin is too tight is that urine sprays all over the place when he passes urine, rather than being in a steady stream. If this happens consistently discuss this with your doctor.

Problems with the scrotum

Any of the structures that lie in the scrotum can become swollen, and these may either be painless or painful.

Painless swelling can be caused by a hernia, which results from a weakness in the muscles of the lower abdomen, and in small boys the swelling may appear to be within the scrotum. I discuss hernias in more detail at the end of this chapter. Alternatively, the swelling may be caused by a hydrocoele, which is a collection of fluid around the testicle. Normally, in the developing foetus there is a connection between the abdomen and the scrotum, and this should close off shortly after birth. However, some of these communications persist and contain fluid, resulting in this painless swelling. Most of these will resolve fully by four years of age. It can be difficult to distinguish between a hydrocoele and a hernia, and your doctor may well refer your son to a surgeon for a full assessment.

If swelling is painful, however, this should always be assessed by a doctor as a matter of very real emergency. The cause may be a torsion, or twisting, of the testicle. This twisting can block the blood supply of the testicle, and lead to permanent damage, so don't hesitate if this is a possibility.

Infection of the epididymis (the tube next to the testicle), the testicle, or even the skin of the scrotum, can all cause pain, but it is so essential that a torsion is not missed that you really do need to let the diagnosis be made by a doctor.

Problems with the penis

Apart from a normal erection, only three things typically damage the penis enough to make it swell. Trauma, infection, and irritation from wet nappies can all make the penis appear abnormally swollen. In addition, hair or cotton twisted around the penis can trap the blood supply and result in a persistent area of swelling and redness after the obstruction. The hair itself may be invisible, merging into the general swelling. As any injury to the penis is potentially serious, seek medical help right away – though the cause may actually turn out to be harmless.

Injuries to the genitals

There are few things more painful than a kick or other injury to the testicles. Boys typically get this injury by falling astride the cross bar of a bike, or something similar. The pain should normally subside after a few hours, but if your child seems to be getting worse, rather than better, there may be bleeding or bruising in the scrotum, and it is worth seeking medical advice.

If your son catches his foreskin in his zip, and it won't come undone easily, then take him right away to a hospital casualty unit where they should be able to deal with it fairly quickly using local anaesthetic. Trying to force the zip along at home can cause increased damage.

Other damage to the skin around the genitals should be dealt with just as you would deal with any other cut or injury. Firm pressure is often all that is required, but be discreet. Remember that your son is likely to be highly embarrassed by such an injury. If you can't stop the bleeding, if the scrotum seems swollen, if pain seems to be increasing rather than getting better, or if there is any difficulty in passing urine, seek medical help.

PROBLEMS WITH GIRLS' GENITALS

Vaginal itching

The skin that lines the vagina is intensely sensitive, especially in small girls. After puberty, the sex hormones lead to the vaginal skin becoming somewhat thicker, and the labial lips become more prominent and act as protection. Before this happens the skin is very prone to irritation by chemicals or other irritants.

Causes

The commonest causes are bubble baths, soap, fabric conditioner, some washing powders, dyes in coloured toilet paper, and so on. In addition, threadworms can cause vaginal as well as anal itching. This topic is covered in detail, on page 144.

When to consult a doctor

If an itch persists and you don't see threadworms, and have tried eliminating all the possible irritants that could be causing the itch, then do seek advice from your doctor. If the itch is associated with discharge, there may be infection present, and I shall deal with this shortly.

Vaginal bleeding

Causes

It is not unusual for a little blood to be lost from the vagina a few days after birth. The cause of this is that the baby's blood at birth contains her mother's sex hormones. As the quantity of these in the blood gradually lessens, a withdrawal bleed – just like a small period – may be triggered off. Providing the bleeding stops right away, then there is no need to do anything else.

When to consult a doctor

Prolonged bleeding, or bleeding occurring at any other time, does need medical attention. Causes can include injury, hormone problems, polyps, and so on.

Vaginal discharge

As mentioned above in the section on vaginal itching, the internal skin of the vagina is very much more sensitive in small girls than it is after puberty.

Causes

A large number of irritants can lead to a vaginal discharge.

These include bubble baths, soap, fabric conditioners, tight clothing (particularly jeans, bodies, or leotards), and foreign bodies in the vagina. Although thrush is a very common problem in teenagers and older women, it is quite rare in children so creams like Canesten tend not to be much help at this age.

When to consult a doctor

If a discharge is persistent, offensive, or bloody then do see a doctor. He or she will almost certainly want to take a swab to find out what particular bacterium is causing the problem. Towards puberty, most girls do lose a little watery, clear discharge as their hormones begin to change. Incidentally, puberty these days can start as young as nine years old.

Obviously if you have any concern at all about the possibility of sexual abuse, then you should seek help immediately. This is still an unlikely cause, but too important to be ignored.

How you can help

Encouraging your daughter to be scrupulous in her personal hygiene may help to prevent future infections. Scratching the bottom and vulval area with dirty fingers is a common childhood activity, but not a particularly good idea! Encouraging your child to wipe herself from front to back after going to the toilet can also help to prevent the spread of bowel germs from the anus to the vagina.

Foreign bodies in the vagina

Causes

Little girls are no better than little boys when it comes to inserting objects into bodily orifices, and little girls have one readily accessible additional orifice to use! Rolled up toilet paper, beads, peanuts, crayons, and almost anything else may be inserted.

When to consult a doctor

A foreign body can act as the focus for infection and this often results in an offensive vaginal discharge. If you can see the foreign body, if it is half protruding, and if it has no sharp edges, then you may be able to get it out. However, if in doubt, don't try. You may push it further inside, and make the problems much worse. It is better to consult a doctor, who will have suitable instruments to sort the problem out, or who may even need to involve a gynaecologist.

If this is a problem that happens just once, don't be worried. If it keeps happening, seek advice. Repeated insertion of a foreign body might be a sign of emotional disturbance, or of sexual abuse.

Problems with the labia

Causes

Until your daughter is about five or six years of age, the outer lips of the vulva may appear to be stuck together. This is a condition known as labial adhesions, and whilst it sometimes might be caused by prolonged irritation or inflammation from nappy rash, it is just as likely to be entirely normal. As your child gets older, the normal increased levels of sex hormones will lead to the adhesions spontaneously breaking down.

When to consult a doctor

Provided your child has no symptoms such as itching, irritation, or bleeding, then leave well alone. Never ever try and separate the lips using force. It can be painful, it is unnecessary, and it won't work. However, if your child does have any symptoms such as discharge which may be aggravated by the adhesions, your doctor may prescribe an oestrogen cream to encourage them to separate naturally.

Injuries to the genitals

Causes

Girls have just the same tendency as boys to fall astride the cross bar of a bicycle – though they are less at risk if they don't borrow a boy's bike and stick to using bikes without the demon cross bars.

When to consult a doctor

If an injury to the vulval area results in any bleeding, I would advise you to consult a doctor right away. In addition, always do this if there is any possibility of the injury penetrating the vaginal entrance, or if your child complains of any difficulty in passing urine after the injury.

SWELLINGS IN THE GROIN

A lump in the groin can be caused by a swollen gland, by a hernia, or by a testicle (or, very rarely, an ovary) that is in the wrong place.

There are normally lymph glands in the groin. These will always swell up if there is any infection in the area. For instance, an infected cut on the leg will lead to the lymph nodes in the groin on the same side swelling up. These help to prevent the infection from spreading further throughout the body. Like the swollen glands that appear in the neck, these should be freely mobile, and firm but not rock hard. If the glands feel very hard, and do not move under the skin, then ask your doctor to check them over. In addition, if the swelling persists for more than a couple of weeks, always seek advice. If there is no testicle present in the scrotum on the side of the body where the lump can be felt, then it is possible that the lump is a testicle that has become stuck in the groin.

A hernia results from a weakness in the muscles of the lower abdomen, through which some of the contents of the abdominal cavity may protrude. As mentioned above, in boys the swelling may lead into the scrotum, but in girls it forms a lump in the groin. A hernia is usually more visible when the child stands up, and may disappear when he or she lies down. This is simply the effect of gravity on the abdominal contents.

Whilst hernias in adults are typically the result of straining for instance from constipation, in children they are usually a result of a congenital weakness. They affect one in a hundred boys, and slightly fewer girls. They only matter if they become strangulated. When this happens, part of the bowel gets trapped in the hernia, and this leads to blockage of the bowel ('intestinal obstruction') and severe pain. For this reason, any hernia in the groin should be repaired to prevent later strangulation occurring. Strangulation is a medical emergency, and you should contact a doctor immediately if there is a hard swelling in the groin that won't disappear and which is associated with severe abdominal pain. A painless hernia that comes and goes is not an emergency, but you should still seek medical advice within a week or so, so that a definite diagnosis and action plan can be made.

The child with an itch

Itching is an extraordinary sensation. Can you really describe it accurately without using the word 'itch'? Itches are, well, itchy. They can also be intensely aggravating and annoying.

Itches can be separated into two separate categories. There are the itches which are generalised and there are the itches that are restricted to one part of the body, for instance the scalp, eyes or anus.

GENERALISED ITCH WITHOUT ANY FORM OF RASH

This is not a particularly common problem in young children, though it can occur. Only last week I saw a little boy who has been scratching for weeks, but after extensive investigations it is beginning to look as if, whatever the initial cause might have been, the problem has now become one of habit.

Causes

Finding the cause of this type of itch is certainly not easy. If your child is taking medication, particularly long-term medication for a condition like epilepsy, then this could be the cause – but please don't stop giving it without seeking medical advice. If necessary initially you could discuss the matter on the phone with your doctor.

Sometimes stress will be the problem, though there is an unfortunate tendency to make stress the diagnosis when all other diagnoses have been ruled out, and this is both illogical, unnecessary, and unkind. Sometimes other medical problems may be causing the itch. Indeed the list of possibilities is too long to go through here.

When to consult a doctor

The simple fact is that a chronic generalised itch is unlikely to be serious, but it could be. So if a significant itch without a rash goes on for more than about twenty-four hours, then please do seek medical advice.

GENERALISED ITCHING WITH A RASH

Frequently itching will be associated with a rash, and I devote a large section of this book to unravelling the different possible forms of rash and their causes. However two vitally important and extremely itchy conditions that I will consider briefly here are urticaria and scabies.

Urticaria (or hives)

Urticaria consists of a raised rash, looking just like nettle rash. Pretty well everyone will develop urticaria if they come into direct contact with nettles. However it has been estimated that nearly five per cent of children will have urticaria from some other cause during childhood. The raised rash is white or almost like a blister, and comes and goes very quickly. It also itches dreadfully.

Urticaria is dealt with fully on page 227.

Scabies

Scabies is another condition associated with a rash

(typically, small red pimples) that causes dreadful itching, and the itch may actually occur a day or so before the rash appears. It mainly affects the skin creases such as the area between fingers, the wrists, and the armpits. It can also affect the abdomen, and in infants the head and neck may be affected as well. The itch is typically worst at night.

Scratching the itch may break the skin. This in turn leads to infection getting into the skin causing the rash of impetigo, which may then make the original cause much harder to diagnose. Impetigo starts as a small pimple, which then rapidly enlarges up to about one inch or more across, forming a blister typically filled with yellow or cloudy fluid. These then break open, the fluid drains away, and a crust forms on the surface. Typically, the area continues to enlarge, and new spots appear nearby. You should certainly consult your doctor about impetigo.

I give a full explanation of the causes of scabies, and the best ways to treat it on page 223. This may tell you more about the life cycle of the scabies mite than you ever thought you wanted to know, but if your family is suffering from scabies, understanding the cause will make treatment far more logical and likely to succeed.

ITCHES IN PARTICULAR AREAS

The Anus

Causes

Probably the commonest cause of pruritus ani in children, the medical term for an itchy bottom, is threadworms. I have given very detailed information about this delightful topic in the section on 'The child with abnormal stools' on page 144.

However threadworms are not the only possible cause.

The area around the anus is often slightly soggy, and this moist skin can become inflamed. This makes the sufferer scratch, the scratch inflames the skin still further, and a vicious circle of scratching and itching is set up.

Many cases of itchy bottom have no other obvious predisposing cause though may be aggravated by poor hygiene (as in the child who is in much too much of a rush to wipe his or her bottom properly when he or she has finished). Sometimes problems such as haemorrhoids or an anal fissure can cause an itch, though haemorrhoids are not common in children, and a fissure is more likely to cause bleeding and pain rather than itching.

Other possible causes of itchiness include nappy rash. This diagnosis should be self-evident, and is dealt with fully in a separate chapter, starting on page 231.

Eczema is another possible cause. You will typically see a patch of dry inflamed skin around the anal area. Your child may also have eczema elsewhere on the body. Eczema is covered in full in the chapter on 'The child with a rash' (page 201) but if an itchy bottom is a major problem in particular you should avoid bubble baths, and even soap. Instead you should use moisturising treatments such as emollients such as Oilatum, Aqueous cream or Emulsiderm, and if necessary hydrocortisone cream.

When to consult a doctor

If the treatment you are trying for your child's itchy bottom does not seem to be working, then do consult your doctor.

Eyes

Causes

Itchy eyes are another very common childhood problem, and are often associated with redness. If your child's eye is indeed red as well as being itchy, then please look at the section in this book on the red eye on page 260. However, if the eyes are itchy, but there is no particular redness then by far the most likely cause is allergic conjunctivitis.

There are two main types of allergic conjunctivitis. The first is hayfever, otherwise known as seasonal allergic conjunctivitis and usually also associated with seasonal rhinitis (or nasal congestion). The other is perennial allergic conjunctivitis. The term 'perennial' simply means that the problems is present all year round.

Either of these may be associated with a blocked nose. They are dealt with more fully in the chapter on allergies on page 238.

When to consult a doctor

With any form of eye problem, you should initially seek your doctor's assessment and advice. Whilst allergic conjunctivitis is a significant nuisance, it is not dangerous and cannot damage the eyes in the long-term. However it is absolutely essential to ensure that you really do have the correct diagnosis.

Scalp

Causes

The commonest causes of an itchy scalp are head lice, dandruff, psoriasis, and eczema. The last three are dealt with elsewhere in this book, and the rest of this section will therefore concentrate on the delightful topic of head lice – one that fills every parent with despair.

Typically, children with head lice complain of itching at the sides of the head and also at the back. The problem is very common, and will affect one child in ten at some time – so there is no need to feel ashamed or guilty if your child happens to be one of the one in ten. There is no doubt that some children do seem to have more trouble than others. However this has absolutely nothing whatsoever to do with cleanliness, household hygiene, being a good parent, or anything else. In fact, head lice actually seem to prefer clean hair.

The lice themselves are spread from person to person by direct contact, or by shared hats, caps, combs, or brushes. They are tiny insects, approximately 3–4mm long, which have such a specialised lifestyle that they only live in and on human hair. However, you will almost certainly never see the lice themselves. What you will see will be their eggs, which are otherwise known as nits.

Nits are white or light pink, and typically are adherent to the hair right where it emerges from the scalp. Nits can be easily confused with dandruff – but don't get dislodged as easily by combing, shaking, or brushing.

When to consult a doctor

If you detect head lice in any of your children, immediately check over the whole family by combing their hair, whilst damp, with a fine-toothed comb. If you do find any signs of live head lice or nits, then treat that person and that person only, but continue to check the rest of the family regularly. Do not treat babies under six months of age without seeking medical advice first.

To get rid of the lice, you use whatever the advised lotion

is for your area. To find out what is currently being recommended have a word with your pharmacist, health visitor, or doctor. Local treatment policies are frequently used to avoid lice developing resistance to several preparations at the same time. If your child has been swimming in the past three days, then wash and dry their hair thoroughly *before* using the treatment. This is essential because chlorine may stop the treatment working. When you have applied the required lotion (such as Derbac M, Suleo M, or Prioderm) allow it to dry naturally without using any form of artificial heat. You should also leave the lotion on for twelve hours, which usually means overnight.

If the lotion has been used properly, all lice and eggs will be dead. They can easily be removed by using a fine-toothed comb on wet hair, or by sliding the eggs off dry hair with your fingernails. It is worth trying to clear the hair of dead lice and eggs as you will then be able to spot a new infestation more easily.

After an infection, it is worth checking the hair weekly by combing damp hair with a fine-toothed comb, and keeping some spare lotion available if live lice or nits are found. However, you should not treat the scalp and hair again 'just for luck' if you do not find live lice again as overuse of these potent medicated treatments is not without risks. Like all medication, they should only be used when strictly necessary.

THE STRUCTURE AND FUNCTION OF THE SKIN

The skin – which is actually the largest organ in the human body – consists of two layers, the epidermis on the outside, and the dermis underneath it. Typically the skin is about 2mm thick, but it tends to be much thicker on the soles of the feet and the palms of the hands than elsewhere on the body.

The skin is an astonishing structure, being protective and waterproof, and healing itself when injured. Its chief function is certainly protective, preventing the other tissues and organs in the body from damage by water, heat, wind, injury, and so on. It also has an important function in regulating body temperature – with sweat glands cooling, and subcutaneous fat preserving heat. It also has a number of other important functions, such as synthesis of vitamin D, but these are less important to an understanding of rashes and other skin problems.

DIAGNOSING RASHES

Most medical diagnoses are reached by a process that is very similar to detective work. The doctor asks a number of questions, looks at a number of clues, tries to piece all these together, and finally arrives at an answer. When unravelling the cause of a rash you can do the same. Sometimes the answer will be obvious – a nettle rash in a child who has just walked through a nettle bed is an over-obvious example – but more often than not you will have to piece various clues together. A chapter like this cannot be a total guide to diagnosis of every rash your child might have, but at the very least I can point you in the right direction.

This section consists of a series of questions. Look at each one in turn. If you answer yes to a question there will be a series of possible diagnoses. If you can only answer yes to one question, then you will probably be left with quite a number of possibilities. But if you answer yes to two or more questions, the diagnosis will become much more obvious.

For instance, if you answer 'yes' to 'Does the rash itch?', and 'Is it worst on the front of the elbows or back of the knees?', but you answer 'no' to 'Does your child have a temperature?', and 'Is your child unwell?', then the likely diagnosis will show up to be eczema.

Incidentally, when diagnosing a rash it really is important to strip your child off and look at the whole skin. Otherwise you will find yourself jumping to unjustified conclusions.

The final part of this section is a more detailed summary of each of the most important skin conditions – though no book this size can ever cover them all.

Does your child have a temperature?

Virus infections, such as measles, German measles, chickenpox; non-specific virus rashes such as coxsackie and echo virus rashes, and roseola infantum; and scarlet fever (not actually a virus!)

Has your child recently had any injections?

A rash may occur about a week after the MMR injection.

Has the rash been present for more than a couple of weeks, or does it keep coming back?

Eczema, psoriasis, fungal rashes

If there is no temperature, does the rash itch?

Eczema, pityriasis rosea

Is the rash confined to one part of the body?

Contact eczema (dermatitis), impetigo

Is the scalp affected – dry, flaky, or thickened?

Seborrhoeic dermatitis, fungal infections, psoriasis, dandruff

Are the feet primarily affected, with a scaly rash on the toes or the ball of the foot?

Eczema, athlete's foot.

Does your child also have a cough?

Measles. If the rash is confined to the area around the eyes, this may come from tiny burst blood vessels from the strain of coughing, and is harmless.

What does the rash look like?

- *Dry skin. Red. Itchy.* Eczema.
- *Distinct separate patches. Dry and Scaly.* Psoriasis, ringworm, eczema, pityriasis rosea.
- *Scaly surface and silvery if you scratch it.* Psoriasis.
- *Flat and under the skin.* Measles, rubella, roseola, allergy rashes, fifth disease, scarlet fever, petechiae, Kawasaki disease.
- *Flat spots, pink or red, with normal skin in between.* Drug reaction or virus infection.

- *Mainly in the form of blisters.* Chickenpox (starts as red spots), herpes simplex (cold sores), impetigo, bites, hand, foot and mouth disease.
- *Only one blister, possibly infected, yellow and crusty.* Herpes simplex, impetigo.
- *Blisters mainly on the hands, feet, and mouth.* Hand, foot and mouth disease.
- *Raised, but not blisters.* Urticaria (nettle rash), erythema multiforme, erythema nodosum, scabies.
- *Tiny white waxy bumps on the skin, often in clusters.* Molluscum contagiosum.
- *In the form of one or more rings, possibly with a clear centre.* Ringworm, pityriasis rosea, Lyme disease.

The individual skin problems covered in this section are (listed in alphabetical order):

Allergic rashes
Athlete's foot
Bites
Chickenpox
Contact eczema
Dandruff and cradle cap
Drug reactions
Eczema
Erythema multiforme
Erythema nodosum
Fifth disease
Fungal infections
German measles
Hand, foot and mouth disease
Herpes simplex (cold sores)
Impetigo
Kawasaki disease
Lyme disease
Measles
Molluscum contagiosum
Petechiae
Pityriasis rosea
Psoriasis
Ringworm
Roseola infantum
Rubella
Scabies
Scarlet fever
Seborrhoeic dermatitis
Urticaria (nettle rash)
Virus rashes such as coxsackie and echo virus rashes

ALLERGIC RASHES

There are two main types of rash triggered by allergy. These are eczema-like rashes caused by direct contact with the skin, which may be localised or generalised, or alternatively a generalised rash that might be triggered off by something taken by mouth.

Contact allergy eczema

Typical things that can cause this are chemicals such as soaps, fabric conditioners, bubble bath, washing powders and so on. If the rash is all over, you may need to do some detective work to find the cause. Biological washing powders are a common culprit, and if your child develops a rash on his feet the first time he wears socks washed in a new 'improved' washing powder, then the diagnosis is perfectly simple and obvious. Sometimes children can seem to become allergic to something you've used for a while, and on occasions it turns out that manufacturers will have changed the constituents of, for instance, a washing powder very slightly – but sufficiently to trigger off rashes in susceptible people.

Sometimes the rash is very localised. This is likely to be a contact allergy. Typical causes are materials such as nickel in a fastening, or the leather or buckle of a watch strap.

With these forms of allergic eczema it is essential to work out what is causing the problem, and eliminate it. If a child is allergic to a washing powder and you keep using that powder, the rash will keep on happening, however many creams and lotions you might slap on.

Once the cause is eliminated, allergic contact eczema tends to respond very well to steroid creams, such as hydrocortisone or Eumovate. Your doctor will be able to advise and prescribe appropriately.

Drug and food allergies

The other form of allergic rash is a generalised blotchy red rash which may well itch. Typically this comes on during a course of medication, in particular antibiotics. Food stuffs may be blamed, in particular shellfish and food colourings. It is important to stop giving whatever is the cause, but I would generally advise checking with a doctor first. Firstly, alternative medication may be needed to replace the drug that your child is allergic to. Secondly, vast numbers of children are diagnosed as having allergies when in fact they simply developed a rash as part of their infection (possibly a straightforward virus infection), but because they are on antibiotics the antibiotics get blamed. Doctors tend to err on the side of caution, but it is likely that tens of thousands of children have their medical records marked as being 'allergic to penicillin' when they are nothing of the sort.

Drug allergies can sometimes take the form of urticaria – which looks like nettle rash, and this is dealt with in its own section.

If allergy rashes are very irritating, these rashes may be helped by anti-histamines or calamine lotion.

Sometimes drug allergies can be much more severe, with not only a rash, but swelling around the eyes and lips and even difficulty breathing, and wheezing. If this occurs seek medical help straight away, and see page 256 of the section on 'The child with allergies'.

ATHLETE'S FOOT

Athlete's foot is one of those poorly named medical conditions. Like tennis elbow, which typically happens to people who have never picked up a tennis racket in their life, athlete's foot frequently happens to couch potatoes and other non-athletes. It is not particularly common in children before adolescence, though appears to be getting somewhat commoner, possibly because of changing trends in footwear. Wearing trainers all the time certainly increases the risk of this condition occurring.

It is a fungal infection of the skin, typically occurring between the toes which become cracked and soggy. The sole and instep may also be affected. The fungus that causes it thrives on warm soggy conditions, so a pair of trainers that don't allow the skin to be ventilated, particularly in warm weather, is a perfect recipe for this condition.

Young children also develop a rash on their feet that may be misdiagnosed as athlete's foot, but which is actually a form of eczema triggered off by the shoes. The actual chemical that your child might be sensitive to could be dye stuffs in the leather, or other chemicals or glues. You can usually tell the two conditions apart because the allergic contact shoe dermatitis does not cause any rash between the toes.

In both these conditions, leaving the feet exposed to the air certainly helps. Athlete's foot can be readily treated with anti-fungal creams or powders. These can be purchased from a pharmacist, or are available on prescription from your doctor. If in doubt about the diagnosis it is important to seek medical advice. Using the wrong type of cream can make things much worse – particularly if you use anti-eczema creams such as hydrocortisone on fungal rashes.

BITES

Many spots seem to be diagnosed as bites, simply because

no other explanation seems to make sense. However, all that looks like a bite is not necessarily bitten.

Flea bites typically occur on exposed areas such as the hands and legs, or on areas where clothing is particularly tight, such as round the waistband. Most fleas spread from pets, but they can survive for many months in furniture or carpets. The most important aspect of treatment is therefore getting rid of the source – by treating carpets, soft furnishings, and your pets.

Insect bites are another common cause of spots. In most families there are people who always seem to get bitten, and others who seem immune. My wife has a dreadful time from insects, but they never seem to touch me. However, and contrary to many people's beliefs, it seems likely that everyone is bitten exactly the same amount. The difference arises in the skin's reaction to the bite. The spots are actually an allergic reaction to the bite, and some people are simply much less sensitive than others.

Typically, bites affect older children, particularly in the summer. Young babies seem nowhere near as sensitive. Generally, a raised white area of skin occurs shortly after a bite, then within a few hours the typical red bite mark spot appears. There are also likely to be several spots within a small area, either in a line or cluster, where the insect has taken bite after bite, enjoying its snack. No particular treatment is needed for these spots and they will gradually fade away over the next couple of weeks. If itching is a real problem, calamine lotion may help, or alternatively a cream called Eurax can be very soothing.

CHICKENPOX

Chickenpox is a very common infectious illness, and it is caused by the virus varicella zoster, which is the same virus that is responsible for shingles. Once a child has had chickenpox then it is extremely rare for it to happen again, and immunity is usually complete. However, the virus may stay dormant in the body for many years and then flare up again as an attack of shingles.

The rash is usually extremely itchy. It typically starts on the body then spreads out to the legs, arms, head and face. Initially the rash starts as raised red or pink spots, then these turn to blisters which eventually burst or crust over to form scabs. Crops of spots keep appearing over about four to five days, and this cropping means that spots in different stages of development may be present next to each other. All the spots will have scabbed over after about five days, but it may take up to a fortnight for them to disappear altogether. Whilst adults with chickenpox tend to feel unwell, for most children it is little more than a nuisance, though they may have a raised temperature.

Chickenpox is infectious from up to five days before the spots appear (when of course you don't know anything about it) until all the blisters have scabbed over. For this reason, most school medical authorities say that children should stay off school for at least five days after the spots first appear or until all the spots become dry.

For the great majority of children, no treatment is needed. However, if your child has any condition which interferes with his or her immunity – for instance if he or she has had recent chemotherapy or radiotherapy – then it is absolutely essential that you seek medical advice right away. In addition, if your child is taking steroids for any reason, then these can make the body's immunity less effective and an injection of immunoglobulin – which will boost the immunity – may be necessary. Without such treatment in someone with poor immunity, chickenpox can become a very serious illness.

Incidentally, if you or your partner have never had chickenpox and you develop it now, then contact your doctor. Adults have a much worse time with chickenpox than children and your doctor may give you an anti-viral drug such as acyclovir. But there is no way that this extremely expensive anti-viral agent is justified in the average child. Finally, if a pregnant woman is exposed to chickenpox it is essential that she discuss this with her doctor right away as there is some evidence that the virus may be hazardous to the developing baby.

Try to persuade your child not to scratch the spots, or pick at the scabs. It might be fun, but it can leave scars or pock-marks. Paracetamol will help if there is a fever, and it is also important that your child drinks plenty of fluids. Calamine lotion will help deal with the itching.

There is some evidence that elderly people are at risk of having shingles activated if they are in close contact with a child with chickenpox.

There is no specific treatment for chickenpox, apart from in the circumstances described above.

There is no immunisation against chickenpox. Indeed the best way to avoid getting chickenpox as an adult is to have had it as a child. If you have an older child who hasn't had chickenpox, there is therefore no reason to keep him or her away from a child with chickenpox – unless getting it would be dreadfully inconvenient, such as immediately before a holiday or even a hospital admission.

CONTACT ECZEMA

See 'allergy rashes'.

DANDRUFF AND CRADLE CAP

Dandruff is much commoner in adults than in children. However a variant of dandruff known as cradle cap is a common problem in infants. The scalp appears thickened and crusty, and either small or large areas of the scalp may be affected. It may be associated with patches of dry scaly skin over the face, and almost anywhere else on the body, known as seborrhoeic dermatitis.

You can loosen the scales on the scalp by gentle daily shampooing, especially if they are loosened overnight with an oil such as baby oil or even olive oil. If the spots are really troublesome, then ask your doctor or health visitor for advice.

With dandruff in children, I think it is best to avoid most of the very strongly medicated shampoos that are advertised for adult use. My impression is that these are actually somewhat more likely to cause dandruff than to cure it in children with sensitive scalps. (Your pharmacist may be able to give you advice on suitable shampoos.) Dandruff is sometimes associated with eczema. If dandruff does not clear up despite washing with gently medicated shampoos, do consult your doctor as it is possible that the cause of the problem is a fungal infection, requiring an anti-fungal shampoo such as Nizoral.

DRUG REACTIONS

See 'allergy rashes', and also 'urticaria'.

ECZEMA

Eczema is sometimes called dermatitis. There is no important difference between the two terms. One word comes from the Greek and the other is Latin.

The main symptom of eczema is dry, inflamed skin. In most children the initial problem is simply dryness, and in mild cases the problem may not become any worse than this. As eczema becomes more severe, the skin becomes more dry and inflamed, with cracking, redness, soreness, itching, or any combination of these.

There are two main types of eczema. Some children develop eczema because either eczema, asthma, or hayfever run in their family. Families in which these three conditions appear are called 'atopic' families. However, it is not inevitable that having one of these problems means you will get the others. In other cases there is a specific trigger or irritation that causes the problem. The child who develops an allergic rash (see the earlier section) has a form of eczema, sometimes known as 'contact dermatitis' or 'contact eczema'.

Eczema can start in infancy, where the whole skin may feel dry, and a rash may appear on the face, scalp, trunk, and outside of the legs and the arms. Typically eczema starts on the face and scalp at some point between three months and two years of age. Black or dark-skinned children may have areas of paler skin, particularly on the face.

In older children the rash primarily affects the fronts of the elbows, the backs of the knees, the neck, the feet, the wrists and the hands – though it may occur anywhere at all.

As well as the rash, itching is a major problem. The child may scratch and scratch, which worsens the rash, which worsens the itch, and one of the most vicious of vicious circles is set up. Scratching releases a chemical in the skin called histamine, and histamine worsens the irritation still further. Even infants may roll their faces against bedclothes in an attempt to ease facial itching.

Eczema can be aggravated by many things. Soap, which

tends to have a drying effect on the skin, is one of the main culprits. Wool or other fabrics may irritate some children. Sometimes diet is relevant, though probably only to a significant degree in about one child in twenty.

Apart from the most minor degrees of dry skin, I believe that every child with eczema should be seen by a doctor, not only to have the diagnosis confirmed but also so that advice can be given on management, and treatment prescribed.

Once you have seen a doctor and treatment has been prescribed, you should certainly return if the rash gets worse, or in particular if any areas become more red, or look inflamed, infected, seem to be spreading, or have crusts or scabs on. In addition, you should always seek help if the itching is preventing your child from getting a good night's sleep.

Firstly, learn as much as you can about the condition. Ask your doctor or health visitor for booklets or information sheets, and, ideally, consider joining a self-help group such as the National Eczema Society which provides a great deal of tremendously valuable and very clear information. The address is in the appendix. Understanding the condition can make a tremendous difference to your child's welfare. Understanding *why* treatments help can help you as well.

It is vitally important to avoid things that dry the skin, such as soap, bubble baths, or baby bath liquids. Even bubble baths that are marketed as safe for children have a tendency to dry the skin and aggravate eczema. You may be puzzled about how you can wash your child if I am suggesting that you don't use soap, but products such as Oilatum or Emulsiderm emollients can wash very effectively whilst simultaneously moistening the skin. Incidentally, don't expect them to produce a lather.

If your doctor prescribes treatment, it really is important

to use this as prescribed – provided that you understand the reason for this and what the benefits are. Many parents shy away from steroid creams, for instance, because they are frightened of side effects. In fact, if you learn about how to use steroids, and how to minimise any side effects, you will feel more in control, and less anxious, and your child will benefit tremendously. In general, using an effective steroid will only be necessary for a short while, and the benefits of using the correct dose greatly outweigh any disadvantages. But using steroid creams haphazardly, without following the instructions, can cause more problems than it solves.

Watch out for things that may be aggravating your child's eczema. Woollen clothes are a typical example. Cotton is much better, and far less likely to be an irritant.

Keep your child's fingernails short. If the eczema is itchy, your child – even the tiniest baby – will scratch it. Scratching can even occur during sleep. Long dirty fingernails in a child with eczema are a perfect recipe for an infection developing in the eczema. In really bad cases of itching, cotton mittens worn during the night can help interrupt the dreadful scratch/itch cycle.

Consider dietary changes if nothing else seems to help. Some children definitely do seem to be worsened by eggs and cow's milk, so it might be worth excluding one or both of these from the diet for a couple of weeks. If this does not make a difference, do not try stricter and stricter exclusion diets which are likely to do more harm than good. Diet is not usually the answer.

Finally, some parents find that hot dry air in centrally heated houses can make dry skin even drier. Humidifying the air by putting a bowl of water near radiators can greatly improve the situation.

It is important to realise that there is no 'cure' for eczema.

Treatment is aimed at control, reducing the signs and symptoms to a minimum. If you go to your doctor for the first time, receive treatment which successfully clears the rash, only to have it return when the treatment is discontinued, this does not mean that the treatment was unsuccessful or a waste of time. This is simply the nature of the problem. It is very tedious to have to continue using treatments, but essential if you are going to minimise the effects of the condition.

I devote an entire section to eczema treatments in section five of this book, detailing how the different types of treatment work and how they should be applied.

What I would like to stress is the importance of using emollients, which soften and moisten the skin. These are the mainstay of treatment, and are particularly helpful when added to the bath water. But beware! A baby bathed in water containing an emollient can be incredibly slippery, and older children might slip when getting out of the bath.

There is some evidence that breast feeding and avoiding the use of cow's milk products reduces the likelihood of a child developing infantile eczema.

The good news is that eczema frequently gets better on its own. Most eczema that starts in infancy has disappeared by the age of ten. Indeed, about fifty per cent of affected children will be free of the condition by the age of six years. This may seem an awfully long time now, but at least it means there is light at the end of the tunnel. Eczema that starts later in childhood is more likely to persist into adult life.

ERYTHEMA MULTIFORME

You may never have heard of this rash, but it is actually quite common. It becomes obvious when the distinct 'target lesions' appear. These are red circles, with a clear ring inside them, and a round red spot in the middle – just like an archery target. Incidentally, erythema multiforme is a typical example of how doctors can make something simple sound complicated. 'Erythema' means 'red', and 'multiforme' means, hardly surprisingly, 'many forms'. So all this term means is that this is a red rash in many shapes and forms.

Typically erythema multiforme starts as spots on the tops of the legs or the arms, and may initially look like a red viral rash or even like urticaria (nettle rash). The rash then slowly changes over four to five days. The red area gradually enlarges, and the centre slowly clears, so you end up with the target lesions.

The rash typically spreads to the palms of the hands, the soles of the feet, the rest of the body, and even the face, particularly the mouth and the ears. The rash can persist for up to a month.

It is usually caused by virus infections, particularly colds, but may be triggered by drugs such as antibiotics. Usually it is just a nuisance, but it may sometimes spread very rapidly and be severe, making the child very unwell. As a result, whilst you may have felt able to diagnose this yourself, I really would advise you to contact a doctor to get the diagnosis confirmed and to have further advice on how it should be treated. If your child seems unwell, or the rash seems to be developing very fast, then get in touch with a doctor right away.

ERYTHEMA NODOSUM

'Erythema nodosum' means 'red lumps'.

Whilst this is quite common in adults, I have only seen it occasionally in children. However, it does occur in children aged over two years, and is an easily diagnosed and quite distinct condition. The child may complain of painful lower legs, and tender red lumps will be seen over the front of one or both legs. They can be painful enough to make your child limp when he or she walks.

Erythema nodosum should be seen by a doctor. It has two main causes. It can be triggered by certain drugs, and there are also a number of other medical conditions that can cause it. By itself, it doesn't need any treatment other than paracetamol for the pain, but the cause needs to be diagnosed, and any treatment will be specific to whatever the cause turns out to be.

FIFTH DISEASE

This curiously named condition got its name from the fact that it is the fifth of the common childhood rashes, after measles, German measles, chickenpox, and scarlet fever. Presumably no one could come up with a better or more descriptive rash at that time, but it does show a distinct lack of imagination.

Fifth disease is caused by a virus known as the parvovirus, and typically attacks children aged between three and twelve years. It is also sometimes known as 'slapped cheek disease', because to begin with, a rash develops on the cheeks which is bright red and looks as if the cheeks have been firmly slapped. The skin around the mouth is not discoloured, and in mild cases the rash may be barely noticeable.

However, during the next phase of the illness a red spotty rash appears on the limbs and trunk. Sometimes this is so fine that it is described as being lacy. The rash comes and goes, sometimes getting worse on exercise, exposure to the sun, or on getting hot, and it may last for a month or even more. However children with this condition tend not to be ill, and there is certainly no need for them to be kept off school. I would go so far as to say that if your child with fifth disease does seem to be significantly unwell, or has a temperature above 101°F, then the diagnosis probably is *not* fifth disease at all, and you should seek medical advice again. The only children who can develop problems with this condition are Afro-Caribbean children with sickle-cell anaemia. This is an inherited blood disease where the red blood cells are an abnormal shape. In the U.K., it affects about one in two hundred black people of West Indian origin, and one in a hundred of West African origin. Typical initial symptoms can be tiredness, headaches, shortness of breath, and jaundice. The diagnosis is made from examining a smear of blood under the microscope.

The only real significance to this virus is that it can sometimes – though not inevitably – affect the unborn foetus. If your child is in contact with someone who is pregnant, do make sure that they know so that the doctor and midwife can be informed.

Fifth disease has an incubation period of between four and twenty days and is known to be infectious before the onset of the rash. It is probably not infectious after the rash appears, but despite this most school medical authorities advise that children with the condition should remain off school until they are clinically well.

FUNGAL INFECTIONS

The chief fungus that causes skin problems is ringworm – a name that often causes parents very real alarm. After all, the very word 'ringworm' makes it sound as if there is a real worm involved – perhaps burrowing in the skin and causing who knows what in the way of mischief. In fact there is no worm of any type whatsoever. The 'ring' describes the shape of the rash, and the 'worm' bit refers to the appearance of the edge of the rash, curled up and looking to someone with an intensely vivid imagination like a worm lying on the skin. The term 'fungus' frequently causes confusion and upset too, with its connotations of mushrooms and toadstools.

Typically, ringworm causes either one or more circular patches of raised red skin, with scaly edges and clear centres. It grows very slowly, and can persist for a very long time. If one ring appears, and then there are suddenly many more smaller lesions all over the trunk, then this is probably not ringworm at all but a rash called pityriasis rosea, which I describe in detail in a later section of this chapter. However I mention it now, as the two conditions are so frequently confused.

The rash can occur almost anywhere on the skin. If it appears on the scalp, then there may also be a circular area of hair loss.

Usually the diagnosis will be obvious on examination, but if your doctor wants to be absolutely certain, or else is in any doubt, then he or she may take skin scrapings. Small flakes of skin will be gently scraped away and sent off to the laboratory where they can be examined under the microscope and the exact fungus – usually a form of tinea – that is involved can be identified and cultured.

Treatment is usually very effective using an anti-fungal cream such as co-trimazole (Canesten), or something similar. These creams can be purchased over the counter, but if they don't seem to be doing the trick, do consult your doctor who will confirm the diagnosis, and may then prescribe stronger creams, or even anti-fungal medication which can be taken by mouth.

Like all fungal problems, ringworm flourishes in warm,

humid conditions. It can be caught from pets – both cats and dogs – and is also quite easily passed from child to child. Transmission is by direct contact – so keep a dressing on the rash if your child is going to school and it is on a potentially uncovered part of the body.

Fungal infections of the scalp can cause what appears to be an itchy form of dandruff. Dandruff in any child aged under the teenage years should make you suspicious of a fungal infection, so do consult your doctor about this. Very effective anti-fungal shampoos such as Nizoral may be used.

Athlete's foot – which I have already described – is another form of fungal skin infection, and the nails may also be affected, usually causing a very thick, yellow, discoloured nail.

GERMAN MEASLES

German measles, otherwise known as rubella, should be slowly dying out. Since the introduction of the MMR vaccine, almost every child now receives immunisation against this condition, but cases do still occur now and then.

The rash is quite similar to that of measles, and is a pinky-red diffuse rash that starts first on the face, and then spreads to the trunk. After the trunk, it spreads to the arms and legs, but almost always by the time it has reached there, it has left the face. I cannot recall seeing a child with rubella who had spots on the face and the arms at the same time.

The other typical sign of rubella is swollen glands behind the ears. However, it must be said that it is terribly difficult for a doctor to diagnose this condition with one hundred per cent certainty. There are so many other virus rashes that look similar to rubella, and the only way a doctor can give a cast-iron guarantee that one particular rash is rubella, is by taking a blood test. As the condition is very mild and generally harmless to the child, this is simply not justified.

However, rubella can cause major problems for unborn children, leading to blindness, deafness, heart disease and other problems. So, if your child is in contact with a pregnant woman, it is essential that she lets her doctor or midwife know straight away. The great majority of women will be fine, as they will already be immune, but it is terribly important that this is checked. Indeed, the whole purpose of rubella immunisation has been to protect pregnant women. Rubella in children rarely needs treatment, other than paracetamol, and almost never causes any complications – although teenage girls can occasionally develop aching joints.

Rubella is infectious for about one week before the rash appears, and for at least four days after this. School medical advisers usually suggest that a child with rubella should stay off school for a week after the onset of the rash.

HAND, FOOT AND MOUTH DISEASE

Every time that I diagnose this condition, I see a look of mild panic or concern flit across the parent's face. So let's make it clear from the start. Hand, foot and mouth disease has absolutely nothing whatsoever to do with the condition known as 'foot and mouth disease' which affects cattle! It is in fact a fairly common condition, caused by the coxsackie virus.

Typically the illness starts with a slight temperature, sore throat, or abdominal pains, though this doesn't happen with everyone. When the rash appears, it looks like tiny round blisters and typically affects the palms of the hands, the tips of the fingers, the inside of the mouth, and the soles and outside edges of the feet. These last for a few days and then fade away, and no particular treatment is required.

Indeed, the only significant problem that children get is the sore mouth which can make eating and drinking very uncomfortable. If this occurs use paracetamol, and some children are able to use a mouthwash – though don't do this if there is a risk that your child may misunderstand the instructions and swallow it!

The incubation period of hand, foot and mouth disease is between three and five days. Children with this are infectious during the period of the illness, and should be kept off school until they are clinically well.

HERPES SIMPLEX (COLD SORES)

Whilst cold sores can occur almost anywhere, the most typical places for them to appear are around the mouth, particularly on the edge of the lips, on the chin, on the nose, and on the fingers or the hand. Typically they look like tiny blisters and are caused by an infection with the herpes simplex virus, type one. This is a completely different virus to the one that causes genital herpes, so do not panic if your doctor diagnoses this in your child.

The word 'herpes' comes from the Greek word meaning 'to creep' and the herpes virus is astonishingly common. Most of the population is known to carry the virus, although not everyone will actually develop cold sores. It has however been estimated that around twelve million people in the U.K. do get repeated attacks – approximately one in five of the whole population – and these unlucky folk can have between two and ten attacks a year.

Typically it causes an eruption of blisters around the mouth and on the lips, about the nose, face and ears, and in the mouth and pharynx. The first infection with this virus may cause a sore ulcerated mouth and possibly a fever, though some infections are worse than others, and some are barely noticeable. This first infection will typically occur in early childhood, for instance after being kissed by a person with the infection. The virus then passes through the skin, travels up a nerve, and hides in a nerve junction until it is later reactivated.

The virus remains dormant in the skin until it is reactivated and flares up in the form of cold sores when the child later has a cold or some other form of upper respiratory infection. In addition the virus can sometimes be triggered by strong sunlight, stress, tiredness, or even skin injury. Before the cold sore actually erupts, the skin may feel rather itchy or tingly, and then the blister or blisters appear. After a couple of days these will crust over, and usually disappear completely in seven to ten days.

Treatment is now available in the form of anti-viral creams such as Zovirax, though these do not completely cure the condition or prevent further relapses. The chief purpose of treatment is to shorten the duration of the actual cold sore and speed up the healing process. In addition, in people who have had previous cold sores, early treatment can actually prevent a full-blown cold sore from developing.

Sometimes the cold sore itself may become infected, and turn into a patch of impetigo. If this happens the blister becomes crusty, yellow and weeping and antibiotics may well be needed. Impetigo is discussed in detail next.

IMPETIGO

Impetigo is a highly-infectious skin condition, caused by bacteria known as either staphylococci or streptococci. Many of us are carriers of these bacteria in our noses, in our mouths, or on the skin, and usually they don't cause any problems at all. However, if the skin becomes cracked or broken, the bacteria can get into the crack and cause red spots that gradually enlarge until they are anything up to 2cm or more in size and turn into fluid-filled blisters. The surface then breaks down, the fluid drains away, the surface crusts over, and new sore spots form and enlarge the original problem. Whilst it typically starts on the face, it can spread anywhere that the child spreads it to. In other words, if your child has an impetiginous spot by his nose, scratches it, then scratches his leg, a fresh spot will appear on the leg.

When the surface of the spot is broken in this way, the condition is highly infectious and outbreaks can go round playgroups and schools like wild-fire. Indeed, children with impetigo should be kept off school for forty-eight hours after antibiotic treatment has been started, unless the spots can be effectively covered. Just about any child can get impetigo. After all, every child gets dirty fingers and picks their nose, or plays in the dirt. (And any child who never plays in the dirt, isn't having a proper childhood!) Parents often think that a diagnosis of impetigo means that their domestic hygiene must be poor, but this simply is not the case.

Your child should always be seen by your doctor, or a nurse practitioner, if he or she develops impetigo, as treatment is usually with antibiotics, either in a cream form or by mouth. Some milder cases may possibly be treated with antiseptic creams instead.

KAWASAKI DISEASE

This ought to be a condition associated with driving high-powered motor bikes, but in fact the condition was first described by a Japanese doctor called Dr Kawasaki. The rash of Kawasaki disease can sometimes be a general red rash that looks similar to that of scarlatina (scarlet fever), or may be more like the rash of erythema multiforme. It tends to be worst over the knees and elbows. However, what makes the condition quite distinctive are the other signs and symptoms which are:

- High fever
- Swollen glands
- Bright red, cracked, sore lips
- A swollen tongue (with a surface like a large strawberry)
- Enlarged and readily visible blood vessels on the whites of the eyes, particularly around the brown or blue area (the iris) – but not associated with pus, discharge, or the other signs of conjunctivitis
- Swollen hands and feet
- Red palms and soles
- Peeling of the skin of the fingertips and ends of the toes (coming on after about a week)

If you suspect that your child may be suffering from this condition, you should very definitely contact your doctor right away. Whilst the majority of cases suffer no adverse effects at all, between ten and twenty per cent of children with the condition can develop a form of heart damage. There is no doubt that early treatment can very definitely reduce this risk. It is likely that your family doctor will ask a paediatrician to see your child straight away if this diagnosis is made, but all this activity is aimed at reducing long-term problems and after effects.

LYME DISEASE

This is a condition that, whilst not common, is certainly important. It is caused by a tick bite, and the tick will typically have come from deer, mice, or occasionally other animals and even humans. Typically children develop this after a camping holiday. The rash looks at first just like ringworm, and consists of a ring that forms around the tick bite, and then gradually fades from the centre, although it can sometimes have a red centre. The chief difference from ringworm is that the appearance changes over a matter of a few days, whereas the changes of ringworm are very much slower. As the bite may well have occurred in the scalp, these changes may remain invisible and unknown.

About a month after the initial bite the child may develop symptoms of flu, and in particular aching in the knees and other joints. It is essential to consult a doctor right away if you even vaguely suspect this condition. It can have serious side effects which can include damage to the eyes and to the heart, but if diagnosed it can be readily treated with antibiotics.

MEASLES

Thanks to immunisation campaigns, this potentially serious illness has now become pretty rare, with only 1,643 cases being reported in England and Wales between July and September 1995, the lowest quarterly figure since 1940 when records began. Internationally, however, it is one of the commonest diseases in the world.

The rash of measles usually starts on the child's face and in particular behind the ears, and it then spreads down over the trunk, the arms, and the legs. The rash is blotchy and very red, and the different patches of spots tend to run into each other.

Many parents suspect their child has measles when he or she develops vague red rashes, but the chief sign of measles is that sufferers tend to be ill. If your child is running around, happy, and otherwise fairly well, it is extremely unlikely that the rash is measles. Typically, children with measles have a high temperature, a fierce barking cough, red or sticky eyes, and in the first couple of days they may have Koplik spots. These are white spots on the mucous membrane on the inside of the mouth, and they may be present before the rash actually appears. The child may actually be vaguely unwell before the rash appears, and an astute doctor may spot the Koplik spots and predict that the rash will appear in the next day or so. Incidentally, some children who have been immunised against measles may develop a milder version of the condition.

The incubation period of measles is between seven and eighteen days, and the condition is infectious from just before the illness starts until four days after the appearance of the rash. The child should be kept off school until he or she is back to normal. Because the disease is now notifiable, and because it may indeed not be measles, you should certainly consult your doctor if you suspect that your child has this condition.

Whilst there is no specific treatment for measles, and the most important aspects of management are keeping your child cool, giving paracetamol, and offering drinks and sympathy, there are a number of possible complications. Some children develop otitis media (a middle ear infection) or a chest infection, and both of these may require treatment with antibiotics – so do have a word with your doctor if your child complains of earache or has a particularly bad and persistent cough.

The most serious complication, which affects approximately one in a thousand cases, is encephalitis – or inflammation affecting the brain. The symptoms of this are headache, neckache, or possibly backache, and in later stages possibly fits. You won't miss this condition. A child with measles encephalitis will be so sick that you won't think twice about calling a doctor.

MOLLUSCUM CONTAGIOSUM

This sounds so much worse than it really is. In this condition the child develops crops of small, smooth, white or skin-coloured, shiny swellings in the skin. They are typically between three and 8mm in diameter, and have a small dimple in the centre. They can occur almost anywhere on the body, but are commonest on the trunk or the buttocks. They are caused by a virus growing in the surface layers of the skin, and are actually similar to a tiny wart – although conventional wart treatments tend to be completely useless.

With no treatment at all, they will eventually disappear. If they are numerous, embarrassing, or unsightly, or if your child simply wants to be rid of them, then do consult your doctor. The traditional treatment is to scratch the top of them, and to apply a chemical known as phenol, although some doctors will also use cryotherapy – freezing them with liquid nitrogen.

Despite the name, they are not particularly contagious except in overcrowded conditions in tropical countries, although it is probably wise for other children to avoid direct contact with the actual lesions.

PETECHIAE

This word is pronounced 'pet-eek-eee-aye' and refers to areas of bleeding in the skin from the capillaries, the smallest blood vessels. The rash itself is made up of tiny discrete bright red dots, which do not disappear when you press on them firmly. The easiest way to examine whether this happens or not is to use a glass to press against the skin. On normal skin, the glass will leave a white mark for a moment and the pinkness will disappear. In petechiae, the spots remain unchanged.

There are a number of possible causes for this condition. Most are not serious, although some are:

- Sneezing, retching, prolonged coughing, or vomiting can produce areas of petechiae on the face. If the face is the only place that is affected, and your child seems to be well in every other way, then there is no cause for concern.
- Being born can also cause petechiae on the face. After all, it is quite a stressful occasion with great pressure being put on the child's facial skin.
- Very tight clothing can cause an area of petechiae in the skin past the area of constriction.
- Virus infections can cause petechiae in two ways. The capillaries themselves may be damaged, or the number of platelets in the blood may be reduced. The platelets are the cells in the blood that clump together to help the blood to clot in case of injury. Every cubic millimetre of blood normally contains an astonishing quarter of a million platelets. When any blood vessel is injured or damaged, the platelets then clump together at the site of the injury and react with other chemicals in the blood known as clotting factors. The combination of the clump of platelets and the clotting factors turns the blood solid in the form of a blood clot. Obviously if any clotting factor is in short supply (as in haemophilia) or if there are insufficient platelets, then clotting will be less effective and bleeding may occur.
- Idiopathic thrombocytopenia is another very important cause of petechiae. 'Idiopathic' always means 'No one knows what causes it', the 'thrombocytes' are the platelets, and 'penia' is the medical term for a shortage. So, idiopathic thrombocytopenia is a shortage of platelets of unknown cause. To make life easier, I will refer to it by its accepted abbreviation of I.T.P. from now on.

- Children with I.T.P. are usually otherwise perfectly healthy, but have low levels of platelets in the blood. This can only be confirmed by a blood test. Frequently it gets better without any treatment at all, but some children may get dangerously low levels of platelets and need admission to hospital, and others may have prolonged episodes and need treatment with drugs such as steroids.
- Meningococcal septicaemia – the rash that accompanies meningococcal meningitis – is a form of petechiae and obviously needs extremely urgent medical attention.

If your child has petechiae and is otherwise well, then you should consult your doctor, though this is certainly not an emergency. However if the petechiae are all over your child's body, or your child seems ill, or has a fever, or the spots are large enough to look like bruises, then you should seek immediate medical attention. Go to the doctor right away, or call an ambulance by 999.

PITYRIASIS ROSEA

This is pronounced as 'pit-eee-rye-assis rose-ear'. It is another rash that I see several cases of each year, and yet I have never met a patient or parent who has ever heard of it. It can occur in small children, though is more common after the age of ten or eleven. It is probably caused by a virus, although no one has yet identified which one. However, the fact that once you get it you won't get it again, strongly suggests that an infection that causes immunity is to blame. Even so, it does not seem to be significantly infectious. I don't think I have ever seen two people in the same family get it, or two children in the same school. So, if it is a virus, it is a pretty unambitious one.

Sometimes the rash appears out of the blue. On other

occasions the patient has the signs of either a cold, or sore throat, or similar viral infection a few days beforehand. The first sign of the rash is a single large oval patch looking very like ringworm, and known as the 'herald patch', occurring on the front or back of the trunk.

Within the next few days, further smaller patches will appear. All of them will be smaller than the herald patch, and typically have a distribution just like a Christmas tree across the back, with the spots facing downwards and out from the centre of the child's back. All of the spots look like ringworm, but the distribution across the trunk, the limbs, the neck, and, less commonly, the face, is unique to this condition.

You should consult your doctor if you suspect this condition, primarily to get the diagnosis confirmed and to be informed that there really is no need to stay off school. Your doctor will probably be marginally astonished if you say that you suspect the diagnosis is pityriasis rosea. There is no treatment, although sometimes the rash can be itchy, and your doctor mighty prescribe anti-histamines or even a mild steroid cream if this is a problem. It will probably last for anything up to two months, but will eventually clear completely.

PSORIASIS

Psoriasis, whilst a common skin problem in adults, is relatively uncommon in children and very rarely affects infants. The rash consists of red patches, with a silvery scaly surface, which hardly itch at all. The places that it appears are almost the exact opposite of the places eczema appears. Whilst eczema occurs on the fronts of the elbows and the backs of the knees, psoriasis tends to affect the fronts of the knees and the backs of the elbows. It also affects the crease between the buttocks, the scalp, the groin, and the area around the genitals. It can also cause pits in the nails, although this is not universal. The main problem that occurs in psoriasis is a considerable increase in the rate at which skin cells divide and grow, and subsequently flake away.

If you suspect the diagnosis of psoriasis, especially if there is a significant family history, then you should very definitely consult your general practitioner to have the diagnosis confirmed. Increasingly effective treatments are now available, in particular in the form of creams, lotions, and shampoos, and as the condition is relatively rare in children it is quite likely that your G.P. may refer your child to a consultant dermatologist for an opinion and advice.

If the diagnosis is confirmed I really would strongly advise you to join the Psoriasis Association, who provide useful and informative material.

RINGWORM

See 'Fungal infections'.

ROSEOLA INFANTUM

This is another common condition that is believed to be caused by a virus, though you might be forgiven for suspecting that doctors seem to blame almost everything on viruses. It typically occurs between six months and two years of age, and starts with a high fever. This goes on for three or four days, and as it settles back to normal a non-itchy, non-specific, reddish rash appears all over the body. It lasts a couple of days, then fades away. One of its characteristic features is the way that the child feels much better as his or her rash appears and the temperature drops. It isn't infectious enough to keep your child away from other children, and rarely needs any treatment other than paracetamol or ibuprofen for the fever.

RUBELLA

See 'German measles'.

SCABIES

Throughout the U.K. there is an epidemic of scabies. It is proving difficult to treat, and no family can consider itself immune. However, parents tend to feel desperately ashamed if their child is diagnosed as having scabies. They feel they must be unclean, uncaring, or bad parents. They are not. Scabies just happens.

It is caused by a mite that burrows under the skin. Too small to be visible to the naked eye, it typically affects the webs of the skin between the fingers and the toes, the back of the hands, the wrists, the palms, and the abdomen, with the head and neck sometimes being affected in infants but rarely in older children. If you look at the skin carefully you will see pimples which are intensely itchy, and with skin-coloured or grey-coloured ridges between three and 10mm long, where the mite actually burrows in.

Scabies has two other main characteristics. It is intensely infectious and intensely itchy, with the itch being particularly bad at night. Children and adults with scabies tend to scratch a lot, and the scratching sometimes leads to infection of the skin in the form of impetigo. Even infants with scabies can scratch. They often rub their hands or feet together or even roll their head on their bedding.

The scabies mite lives only on human skin. The female mite is fertilised on the surface of the skin, and then burrows into the skin to find somewhere to lay her eggs. The eggs take four days to hatch, and about ten days later the mature mite appears on the surface of the skin.

The itching is actually caused by an allergy to the mite, the eggs, and the larvae. It may even begin a couple of days before the actual rash breaks out. It is most severe at night or when the skin is warm, but symptoms may take anything up to a month to develop after a person is infected with the mite. The inevitable result of this is that a child can pass the infection on well before anyone is even vaguely aware that he or she is infected at all. The mite itself can be spread by close physical contact, and in particular sharing beds or items of clothing. The mite, in fact, can only live for up to four days away from human skin, so clothes or fabrics that have not had contact with human skin for more than four days cannot harbour any live mites.

If you diagnose scabies in your child, do contact your doctor, health visitor, or school nurse for advice. They will give you advice about what treatment to use, or provide a prescription for a suitable lotion such as Lyclear (permethrin 1%) Quellada (lindane), benzyl benzoate, or gamma benzene hexachloride which should kill the mites. There is an increasing national problem of resistance to the standard treatments, so it is possible that two or more preparations might be needed before complete cure is achieved.

When applying the relevant lotion, you must apply it to the whole body. In particular, pay special attention to the webs of the fingers and toes and to brushing lotion under the ends of the nails. In the case of children aged under two years, you should also apply the treatment to the scalp, neck, face, and ears. In older children and adults, you just apply the lotion up to the neck – unless previous treatment has failed – as scabies rarely affects older children above this point. Usually one treatment will be enough to eradicate the mite, but it is quite common for the itch to persist for some weeks after the infestation has been eliminated. If this is the case you can use a cream like Eurax hydrocortisone (crotamiton), calamine lotion, or even oral anti-histamines.

However, it really is important to treat the entire family. The condition is extremely contagious, and it is possible to have an infestation with the mite well before any signs or symptoms appear. It is therefore totally illogical to treat the affected member of the family alone, as another family member may be a time bomb waiting to re-infect your child again shortly. So, however much other family members might object (or however much you object yourself!), you should all be treated. Do follow the instructions on the preparation carefully, and at the same time as treating everyone in the family make sure that you launder all the clothes and bedding that you have been using over the past four days.

SCARLET FEVER (SCARLATINA)

At last! An infection that is *not* caused by a virus. Scarlet fever, or scarlatina, is caused by a bacterium known as the streptococcus. Commonest in children before the teenage years, it can also occur in adults, and the same bacterium can also cause tonsillitis, impetigo, and sore throats.

Typically it starts with a severe sore throat, and then after a couple of days the body becomes covered with a rash made up of tiny spots that can feel somewhat coarse rather like sandpaper, and which turn pale when pressed firmly. The rash begins on the neck and the chest, and subsequently spreads to the whole of the body, although it tends to be worse along skin folds, in the groin or armpit for example.

Whilst some children get this very mildly, some may be very ill with a high fever, vomiting, a red and flushed face but with pallor around the mouth, a white-coated tongue with red patches known as a strawberry tongue, and even peeling of the skin as the rash clears.

This is an infection that should always be treated with antibiotics – usually penicillin – because it does carry a risk of causing complications such as ear infections, inflammation of the kidneys (nephritis), or rheumatic fever. The antibiotics probably don't make much of a difference to the scarlet fever itself, but they will certainly help to prevent these potentially major complications. I must stress that almost everyone does recover from the condition without any significant complications at all.

Apart from antibiotics, the treatments are the same as for any of the other similar feverish infections – namely plenty of fluids, paracetamol, and lots of sympathy. As yet there is no immunisation available against this condition. The incubation period of scarlet fever is between one and three days, and it is infectious until the sufferer has been on an appropriate antibiotic for forty-eight hours. It is generally recommended that children with this condition are kept off school or away from playgroups or toddler groups until forty-eight hours after the treatment begins.

SEBORRHOEIC DERMATITIS

This is a common form of eczema, and despite its name it has nothing to do with sebum, or any form of greasiness. Its commonest manifestation in children is as cradle cap, which I dealt with fully earlier in this chapter. However, it can also affect the rest of the skin apart from the scalp.

There are two quite distinct types of seborrhoeic dermatitis, the adult form and the infantile form. I shall only deal with infantile seborrhoeic dermatitis here. It affects young children in the form of a florid red skin eruption, with well-defined lesions on the trunk, and areas in the skin creases (such as the groin) which run together, associated with scaling of the scalp. Unlike the other main form of eczema, atopic eczema, seborrhoeic eczema does not itch.

The good news is that typically it clears in a few weeks and seldom recurs. Children who have had seborrhoeic eczema are no more likely than any other child to suffer from the adult form.

URTICARIA (NETTLE RASH)

The old name for urticaria was 'hives', and its appearance is exactly the same as the appearance of the skin when stung by nettles. Anyone can experience urticaria if they have put their hand into a nettle bed, but if you've been lucky enough never to experience a nettle sting, then the appearance is of a swollen and raised area of pale skin, surrounded by a red weal. These weals can appear anywhere on the body and may vary in size from being just a tiny spot to a large patch many centimetres across. The rash changes in appearance very rapidly. It typically comes on suddenly, and can come and go in a matter of minutes. Individual weals typically only last a few hours, but others will meanwhile be erupting at other sites. After it has faded away it may leave a faint blue colour to the skin that then disappears completely over the next few days. Urticaria is remarkably common in children aged under five, and it has indeed been estimated that nearly five per cent of children will have urticaria from some other cause during childhood. It can occur at any age, and frequently no cause will ever be found.

When a cause can be identified, the most likely culprits include foods (such as eggs, nuts, chocolate, cheese, fish, sweet corn, pork) and food colourings and food additives (such as tartrazine [E102], monosodium glutamate, and others). When foods are the cause this can be very obvious. I well remember being called to a young patient of mine who was covered in urticaria within minutes of being fed a boiled egg, but sometimes there will be a delay of several hours before the reaction. However, don't ban your child from a foodstuff on a hunch – unless the reaction was very severe, or it occurs on more than one occasion after a particular food. It would be terribly sad if your child spent a lifetime avoiding a particular food that was actually completely harmless!

Drugs are another common culprit, in particular anti-biotics such as penicillins, although almost any drug can be the cause. It must be remembered that people can become allergic to something that they have had perfectly safely and with not a hint of an ill effect for several years.

In other children the trigger can be exercise, streptococcal infections, pressure on the skin, heat, sunlight, and so on. You can see why it can be a nightmare trying to unravel the cause.

Frequently children will have a single attack of urticaria, for it never to return again, and if this is the case then knowing the cause, whilst interesting, is largely academic. For children in whom the problem keeps returning, you have a bigger problem and you will need to return to your doctor to discuss the options.

Sometimes urticaria will be associated with difficulty in breathing – typically wheezing – or swelling of the eyelids or lips. This is a condition known as angio-neurotic oedema (with the neurotic bit having nothing to do with its rather derogatory lay meaning), and you should seek medical advice immediately. Your doctor will almost certainly give immediate anti-histamine treatment, plus possibly adren-aline by injection and possibly steroids.

The mainstay of the treatment of urticaria is anti-histamine medication as syrups or tablets. These are dealt with fully in the appendix to this book on different drugs. When choosing an anti-histamine it is generally best to opt for one of the newer non-sedative types such as terfenadine (Triludan). The older ones (Piriton – chlorpheniramine) were much more sedative, which can be a significant nuisance for some children, and essential for others who simply can't get to sleep because of the intensity of the itch. Such sedation may sometimes be helpful.

On rare occasions urticaria becomes and remains a very major long-term problem. My own daughter has suffered from a type known as exercise urticaria for very many years, and she will tell you right away that the massed brains of the best doctors we could find for her singularly failed to make any difference to it whatsoever. Thank heavens that such therapeutic failure is a relative rarity!

VIRUS RASHES SUCH AS COXSACKIE AND ECHO VIRUS RASHES

Unfortunately, whilst many of the rashes that I have described in this section are absolutely distinctive – the rashes of pityriasis rosea and chickenpox being two good examples – many children develop rashes that are extraordinarily difficult to label accurately. Many of these are rashes associated with other virus infections, typically those caused by the coxsackie and echo viruses. These rashes are typically flat, red, and may remain separate or can blend in together. They tend not to itch, and usually when you press them the rash blanches (unlike the rash of petechiae). The rashes are infuriatingly similar to the rashes caused by drug allergies, and as many children will be taking antibiotics (possibly well meaningly but unnecessarily) for these virus infections when the rash appears, it can be difficult to know if the cause was the virus or the antibiotic. As a general rule, allergic rashes are much more likely to itch than virus rashes.

Apart from paracetamol, if the child is feverish or has any discomfort, simple virus rashes require no specific treatment.

The child with nappy rash

There can be few medical conditions more accurately or obviously named than nappy rash. Whilst it is a tremendously common problem, it can certainly be extremely sore and uncomfortable for the child. In addition, it often causes parents concern because they feel that they must be doing something wrong to cause the rash to develop. Concern then gets muddled up with feelings of guilt and incompetence – an all-too-common sensation for parents!

There can be very few children who never ever get nappy rash. Indeed, sometimes it can be a real puzzle. You can put your child to bed and his skin is perfect, but on waking the skin appears to be red and sore. Most frustrating! And there is no doubt that some babies do have more sensitive skin, just like adults.

Symptoms

The term 'nappy rash' simply describes any rash in the area covered by a nappy. The skin can be inflamed, weeping, even bleeding. The area round the anus is very often sore in children with loose stools, and breast-fed babies do naturally have looser motions.

Causes

Nappy rash often used to be called ammoniacal dermatitis because it can be caused by the effect of the ammonia in stale urine on the skin leading to inflammation and soreness. In the folds and creases of the buttocks where urine doesn't reach the skin is much less likely to be affected.

One of the mysteries of nappy rash is not the fact that it happens so often, but that it doesn't happen all the time. After all, the recipe of soggy skin, that becomes warm, and may be cracked, is perfect for bacteria getting in, thriving and multiplying.

Babies between the ages of nine months and a year pass a remarkable volume of urine. This can result in the nappy becoming more wet than its absorbency can deal with. Soreness then develops around the waist, and the top of the thighs, where the nappy edge can rub the skin.

Nappy rash is also caused by infection, of which the commonest form is thrush, a type of yeast also known as candida albicans. Thrush lives on most people's skin all the time. If, however, the skin gets wet or sore, its normal effective protective barriers can become less effective, and infection takes hold. The infection then spreads into skin folds and creases – so distinguishing this rash from ammoniacal dermatitis which tends to spare these areas. Thrush is likely to be present in any rash that's been present more than a couple of days and may be associated with a thrush infection elsewhere in the body. Satellite spots, which are small areas of sore redness that are slightly away from the main area of nappy rash, are also very common. Thrush is, somewhat surprisingly, often not particularly uncomfortable for the baby.

A much less common cause of nappy rash is psoriasis. Usually there will be a history of this in the family. Typically the rash is scaly, and will often be present elsewhere on the body.

When to consult a doctor

Consider seeing your doctor if:

- The rash is not clearing despite normal treatments
- It is particularly severe
- There is bleeding
- You suspect an infection with thrush
- There are fluid-containing yellowish blisters. These could be caused by an infection by the staphylococcus bacteria, and will need antibiotics
- The rash spreads elsewhere, other than just the nappy area

How you can help

Perhaps the best, and certainly the easiest, way you can help is by leaving your baby's nappy off for a while. I know that this isn't always terribly practical, especially if you value your carpets, but it really can help, particularly if the skin can be exposed to warm dry air.

- Always dry your baby's skin carefully when washing and after changing.
- Use barrier creams – such as zinc and castor oil – which can help to protect against the effects of the ammonia.
- If you are one of the few parents who still use terry nappies, use one-way nappy liners which can make a remarkable difference.

Treatment

Your doctor will treat nappy rash with a cream such as 1% hydrocortisone cream, for an uninfected rash, or possibly an anti-fungal cream, or combination cream that contains a mild steroid and anti-fungal agent.

If you are certain of the diagnosis you can buy creams such as 1% hydrocortisone or co-trimazole (Canesten) from a pharmacist.

Prevention

The most important secret to preventing nappy rash is dryness. Keep the skin of the nappy area as dry as you can. Disposable nappies certainly help with this. When you take a nappy off, flush the contents down the toilet, tape up the nappy, and put it out in a bin liner right away. If the nappy is only partly soiled, please don't try to save money by drying it out and re-using it. This is something I have known happen on many occasions, and for families on a low income it is understandable, but it is also a recipe for rashes.

If you are using terry nappies, then impeccable hygiene is absolutely essential. When a nappy is dirty, flush the contents down the toilet, and rinse the nappy clean in the water that is flushing into the toilet. Put the nappy immediately into a plastic bucket which you need to keep ready full of nappy sanitising solution. Make sure that you follow the instructions on the packet, and that the bucket has a lid – especially if you have a toddler! Wash nappies each day, using very hot water, and rinse them very thoroughly indeed. It is also wise to avoid both biological washing powders and fabric conditioners, as either of these can cause skin irritation in small babies.

Quite simply, keep the skin as clean and dry as you possibly can, but despite your best intentions, you must accept that you can't always prevent nappy rash.

The child with a verruca or wart

Symptoms

Perhaps the most important thing to make clear about warts and verrucas is that there is no difference between them. Traditionally, a wart on the sole of the foot is called a verruca, but it is still just a wart. It is not terribly serious and, typically, it is just a nuisance.

Warts cause a lump to form in the skin, and in most children that is the end of the story. They are usually not painful, but warts on the soles of the feet may become painful simply because the body's weight is being put on the verruca each time the child walks. In addition, warts can sometimes become infected, and when this happens they may well be painful.

The commonest places for warts to appear are on the feet, on the hands, and on the fingers – particularly around the fingernails. In older schoolchildren who write a lot, a wart that occurs just where a pen or pencil is gripped may also become uncomfortable, simply because of the pressure that is exerted on it in that position. Warts may occur singly, or – on the feet in particular – there may be a cluster of what are described as mosaic warts, which are given that name for obvious reasons.

Warts can also occur around the anus or on the genital area. In children this is not something that you should ever attempt to treat yourself. It really is important that you seek your doctor's advice if your child develops such warts.

Causes

Warts are caused by a virus, known as the human papillomavirus (HPV), that gets into the skin. It is a much slower acting virus than the typical virus that causes colds and flu, but is just a virus all the same. Warts cannot be caught congenitally, so if a newborn baby has what appears to be a wart then do consult your doctor, as it is likely to be something else. Almost all children will develop a wart at some time. Left alone, almost all warts will disappear spontaneously when the doctor has built up the necessary immunity to the virus. About fifty per cent of warts disappear in six to twelve months without any treatment at all.

When to consult a doctor

Consult your doctor if you have any doubts about the diagnosis of what you think is a wart, if it is on the genital area, if it is painful, or if it is unsightly (for instance a wart on the face). If you are certain that your child has a wart and it is painless, then it does not need to be treated. If you aren't worried, and your child isn't worried about it, then neither is the doctor.

Treatment

Warts that are painful or unsightly and which need treatment are typically first treated with over-the-counter or on-prescription wart removers. These are paints, gels, or plasters containing chemicals such as salicylic acid, podophyllin, or glutaraldehyde.

If these have been tried and the wart is still persisting and painful, then cryosurgery can be used to remove them. Cryosurgery involves freezing the wart. It has been in use, in one form or another, for many years, but modern techniques involve the use of liquid nitrogen, which can be sprayed or touched onto the wart. In effect, this treatment is actually a carefully controlled cold burn. The procedure is somewhat uncomfortable, which is why most doctors are reluctant to carry it out on very young children. It lasts just a very few seconds, and afterwards redness and swelling may appear over the wart, and even blistering is not uncommon. Cryosurgery is, however, extremely effective and it may be available from your G.P., or you may need to be referred to your local dermatology department.

As an alternative to cryosurgery, some doctors will also remove the wart under a local anaesthetic using techniques such as electrocautery or curettage. However, as all these procedures can be painful it seems completely illogical to use them for a condition that is painless. This is the chief reason for restricting treatment to painful warts, especially in children.

Prevention

There is no simple and practical way to prevent warts. Certainly, insisting that children with warts and verrucas either do not swim, or keep them covered with special socks or dressings is now known to be a complete waste of time. Almost all school medical officers now say that such precautions are unnecessary. A few teachers still seem to get upset by the sight of a verruca, and if this is the case it is tactful and simple to cover it with a waterproof plaster, but from a medical point of view most doctors would now think that this is valueless.

The child with allergies

In recent years, allergies have been blamed for everything under the sun. Whether it is bad behaviour, sleep problems, inattentiveness, runny noses, or almost anything else, someone somewhere will put it all down to an allergy. The simple fact is that most of these so-called allergies are nothing of the kind.

Frequently when people talk about allergies, they are actually referring to 'intolerance' rather than true 'allergy'. This is not splitting hairs. There is a fundamental difference between the two different concepts. It is essential to understand what the various terms mean if you are to make any sense at all of articles that you read, or of talks and broadcasts that you might hear.

So, what is an allergy? Whenever a potentially harmful chemical comes into contact with the body, the body's defences immediately produce protective chemicals. This happens with all of us. However, in an allergic person the body mistakes a usually harmless substance for a harmful one and the protective reaction occurs inappropriately. Any substance that triggers this reaction is called an allergen, and the range of possible allergens is vast – ranging from pollens, through mites that are found in house-dust, to drugs or foods.

The majority of children with allergies inherit this tendency. If both parents have allergies, there is a two out of three chance that their children will have allergies. If one parent has allergies and the other does not, then the children have a twenty-five to fifty per cent chance of being allergic, and if neither parent has allergies the risk for the child is around ten per cent. Incidentally, the children of allergic parents do not necessarily have the same type of allergy as their parents.

However, even if a child is allergic he or she won't have any symptoms until he or she has been exposed at least twice to the substances to which he or she is allergic. On the first exposure the body may develop antibodies to the substance. These are very similar to the antibodies produced when the body is invaded by a virus or bacteria. In the case of allergies, the particular antibody is an immunoglobulin called IgE. These antibodies are found in the lining of the nose, throat, lungs, skin, and gut. When the allergen and the antibodies come into contact with each other, another chemical – histamine – is released from cells known as mast cells. This dilates, or opens up, the blood vessels and makes their walls more porous.

As a result of this, normal tissue fluid leaks through the blood vessel walls and if the allergy is in, for instance, the nose, then the lining of the nose swells up, the nose runs, and so on. If the problem is in the lungs, an attack of asthma may be triggered. In the skin urticaria, or hives, may be the result, and in the bowel symptoms such as nausea, vomiting, abdominal pain and diarrhoea may occur, and sometimes nasal and chest symptoms might be triggered off. Whichever part of the body produces the symptoms is known as the target organ.

The main parts of the body where allergies cause problems are:

- The nose
- The eyes
- The skin
- The gut
- The lungs

In addition, a very major form of allergic reaction known as anaphylactic shock can occur and is discussed fully at the end of this chapter.

This chapter will look at each of these particular problems in turn, but you will have seen from this introduction that the basic principle behind all these conditions is very similar.

THE NOSE

Any medical condition that is connected with the nose is likely to be described using the term 'rhino'. A plastic surgery operation on the nose is technically a 'rhinoplasty'. A runny nose goes by the delightful term 'rhinorrhoea', and inflammation in the nose is 'rhinitis'. Allergies cause rhinitis, and are split into two main groups – perennial rhinitis, and seasonal rhinitis. Gardeners will be well aware of the word 'perennial', but the thesaurus describes it as 'constant', or 'long lasting'. Perennial rhinitis continues all year round, whilst seasonal rhinitis just occurs in one particular season. This is more commonly known as hayfever.

Symptoms

Hayfever is a condition that chiefly affects the nose and the eyes. It is actually relatively uncommon in babies and toddlers, but is increasingly common in older children. The main nasal symptoms are sneezing, a constantly runny or congested nose, an itching nose, and also watering and itchiness of the eyes. However, I will deal with the eye symptoms in a separate section. As with so many other medical conditions, the word hayfever is almost totally inappropriate. After all it is almost never anything to do with hay, and it certainly doesn't cause a fever. Perennial rhinitis causes just the same symptoms, but with no seasonal pattern.

Causes

Allergic rhinitis tends to run in families, and is generally commoner in teenagers than younger children. Seasonal rhinitis occurs each year during the same season, and is caused by an allergy to certain grasses, trees, or weeds. These are the plants that depend on the wind for cross-pollination and which therefore release their pollen into the air. Pollen allergies typically occur in the spring and early summer.

Perennial rhinitis can be triggered by allergy to almost anything that is present year-round, but the most common triggers are house-dust or house-dust mites, animals, birds, moulds, chemicals, or plants. Sometimes no obvious cause can be found. If it turns out that your child is allergic to house-dust or house-dust mites, please do not take this as an attack on your standards of household cleanliness. Dust is everywhere. Have you ever noticed the incredible amount of dust in the air if you shake the bedclothes in a room where the morning sun is streaming in through the window? Dust is a fact of life, although there are things that you can do to damp it down. Indeed, it has been calculated that as we breathe, we take in particles of vegetable or animal matter from about 350 cubic feet of air every twenty-four hours.

Similarly, children can become allergic to a pet that you may have had for years. You may get a clue to this if your child seems to get better when out of doors, or well away from the pet – for instance when he or she is at school.

When to consult a doctor

Whilst hayfever treatments can be purchased over the counter at pharmacies, I do think it would be well worth consulting your doctor if your child appears to have either seasonal or perennial rhinitis. The doctor will be able to make a full assessment of the possible causes of the problem, may be able to provide information sheets, and can prescribe treatment which will therefore be free for children aged under sixteen.

Occasionally, the doctor may feel it worthwhile to arrange skin tests to try to pinpoint the exact cause for your child's allergy, but this is certainly not always essential or indeed particularly helpful, in that it may well not change the way that you choose to manage the problem. Most doctors nowadays will not suggest these. In the past, they were used much more frequently as there was the possibility of desensitising injections. This was a course of injections, in which the person with the allergy was initially given an extremely dilute strength of the allergen as an injection, and then the concentration was gradually and slowly built up until immunity was improved. Whilst these could work, and many people had courses of injections such as Pollinex, they carried a genuine risk of triggering a full-blown anaphylactic reaction and even the occasional death. No one dies of hayfever. The treatment was much worse than the illness. As a result, desensitising injections are now only ever used if there is full resuscitation gear to hand, including cardiac defibrillators. Only the very worst allergies justify this level of risk.

How you can help

There are a number of ways that you might be able to help

prevent episodes of rhinitis, and I shall deal with these shortly. However, two other things may be particularly helpful. Make your house a no-smoking zone. There is absolutely no doubt at all that smoke worsens the symptoms of rhinitis, and if you or any other adults must smoke, then at least go into the garden (or even behind the bike sheds!).

Secondly, if your doctor does prescribe or recommend medication, do make sure your child receives this regularly. It can be tempting to discontinue the treatment the moment your child seems to have improved, but many therapies do require relatively long-term treatment.

Treatment

There are different logical ways that treatment might work:

- You could ensure that your child never comes into contact with the allergen – the thing that he or she is allergic to
- You could damp down the inflammation in the lining of the nose
- You could attempt to prevent the release of histamine
- You could try and reverse the effects of histamine after it has been released

All these approaches are possible, although some are much easier than others. For instance, if you know for certain that your child is allergic to fresh flowers during the pollen season, then you don't bring fresh flowers into the house. However, if you know that tree pollens cause the problem, there is not a lot that you can do other than move to the Alps and live above the tree line, or enclose your child in a goldfish bowl so that pollen never comes into contact with his nose. And even more tricky is the decision that you make if you discover your child is allergic to your much-loved family pet. Saying goodbye to the pet could cause more harm than any amount of sneezing, and need for medication. But these are very personal decisions which every family has to make for itself. I will shortly return to ways in which you can reduce the impact of some allergens on your child's life.

Reducing inflammation can be achieved very successfully using nasal sprays that contain a very tiny dose of steroid. This is the basis of drugs such as Beconase, Syntaris, or Flixonase. They have to be used on a regular daily basis, but can be extremely effective. Most are given twice daily, but the more expensive Flixonase can be used once a day.

An exception is the use of disodium cromoglycate nasal sprays which can be very effective in blocking histamine release. The most used brand is Rynacrom, and this is an identical drug to Intal, which is often used for treating asthma in children. It needs to be used between two and four times daily.

There is no evidence of significant problems resulting from the long-term use of these nasal sprays, although most other forms should certainly not be used long-term.

Finally, and probably the mainstay of treatment for most children, are the anti-histamines. The great advantage of anti-histamines is that they deal with all aspects of the allergy throughout the body. So, if your child has eye symptoms as well as nose symptoms, the same medication will frequently deal with both conditions.

The older anti-histamines tended to be rather sedative. These included drugs such as Piriton (chlorpheniramine), Phenergan (promethazine) and Optimine (azatadine), but the more modern equivalents – such as Triludan (terfenidine), Hismanal (astemizole), Zirtek (cetirizine), and

Clarityn (loratidine) – are much less likely to have significant side effects.

Many children start with one approach, such as an anti-histamine, and only add or substitute other therapies if this does not seem to be working sufficiently well. However some children who suffer more than most might need an anti-histamine, a steroid nasal spray, and disodium cromoglycate eye drops. Thank goodness that this is unusual.

Incidentally, there is no cure for hayfever, although many children will typically grow out of it within about ten to twenty years.

Prevention

If you know what the allergen is, then it makes sense to avoid it, but I have already pointed out the very real problems that this can cause. However, you may be able to minimise the problem in a number of ways:

- If possible, get rid of any old or musty furniture that may be harbouring dust, mould, or dust mites
- Vacuum clean soft furnishings, carpets, rugs, and mattresses frequently
- Consider mattress covers that are designed specifically to help keep dust down
- In the bedroom, use foam rather than feather pillows, damp dust the room every two or three days, and try and avoid clutter in the room. In the average child's bedroom this will be an interesting challenge!
- Consider persuading your pets not to come into the main living areas
- Avoid toys that might collect dust and cannot be washed

THE EYES

The basic principles of allergy are exactly the same for the eyes as they are for the nose, and the problem should be approached in just the same way.

Symptoms

Allergy affecting the eyes causes a condition called allergic conjunctivitis. The main symptom is swelling of the lining of the eyelids, watery eyes, and tears may run into the nose and cause nasal swelling and blockage.

Causes

The delicate membranes that line the eyes and eyelids contain a great many mast cells, which you will recall are the cells that release histamine. Antigens coming into contact with these cells trigger the release of histamine, and result in swelling and streaming. The antigens tend to be the same as those which can cause allergic rhinitis.

When to consult a doctor

With any form of eye problem, you should initially seek your doctor's assessment and advice. Whilst allergic conjunctivitis is a significant nuisance, it is not dangerous and cannot damage the eyes in the long-term. However, it is absolutely essential to ensure that you really do have the correct diagnosis.

How you can help

The advice on how you can help allergic conjunctivitis is

identical to that given in the section on allergic rhinitis. In summary – don't expose your child to tobacco smoke, try to avoid potential allergens if this is possible, and ensure that any eye drops are used regularly.

Treatment

The mainstay of treatment for allergic conjunctivitis is disodium cromoglycate. This acts on the mast cells to prevent histamine release, and can be extremely effective. The most commonly used proprietary brand is Opticrom, though there are a number of other alternatives available. Although they are all free of side effects, they do all have a slight disadvantage in that they have to be used four times a day. More recently a newer drug called Rapitil (nedocromil sodium) has been introduced which works in the same way but may only have to be used twice a day.

Prevention

The general advice I gave in the section on allergic rhinitis holds equally true for allergic conjunctivitis. Some people find that dark glasses help, but this obviously depends on the age of your child.

THE SKIN

Both allergy rashes and urticaria are dealt with fully in the chapter on 'The child with a rash' (page 189).

THE GUT

Few topics in childcare cause as much controversy as allergies to food and to food additives. On the one hand certain self-help groups claim that a majority of childhood behavioural problems result from food and chemical allergies and intolerance, while on the other some of the more conservative paediatricians dismiss the topic almost completely.

One of the great difficulties in any discussion of food allergy is that different people often use the same words to mean different things. Take the word 'allergy' for instance. Many reactions that children might have to food are not true allergies at all. I have already explained the biochemical basis of allergies, but the question of why particular allergies occur is something of a mystery, although there is some evidence that exposing babies to particular foodstuffs too early in life may be part of the problem.

Throughout our lives, the walls of our intestines allow certain nutrients to pass through, keeping others in the bowel. In early infancy the bowel is less selective. Large proteins can pass through the bowel wall in the first three or four months, proteins that are up to ten times as large can just about pass through at four to six months. These proteins may lead to antibody formation, and to full allergic reactions when the child is later exposed to these foodstuffs again. If the introduction of the food had been delayed till after six months of age, its proteins would not have passed through the bowel wall, the antibodies would not have been formed, and the allergy might not have occurred. Though still only a theory, this is plausible enough to constitute yet another argument to delay weaning, and mothers who have allergies would be wise to breast feed for as long as possible – avoiding cow's milk 'top-ups' if they can.

Symptoms

So, how do you tell if your child has a food allergy? Listed below are some of the conditions that have sometimes been associated with these allergies to foods. Please do remember that all these symptoms have many other possible causes, and allergy is only one. However, there are certain hints that will help you spot if allergy is a likely problem. For a start it is essential to realise that if a particular symptom is caused by a food allergy it will occur on every occasion your child eats that food. If it only occurs sometimes, it is not an allergy.

Childhood conditions that may be linked to food allergies

Eczema
Hayfever
Asthma
Migraine
Abdominal pains
Diarrhoea
Acute swellings of mouth or tongue
Urticaria
Vomiting
Bloated stomach
Conjunctivitis
Recurrent cough
Runny noses
Ear Infections
Acute anaphylactic shock (the most serious, but mercifully rare)

Sometimes the answer as to whether your child has a food allergy will be obvious. If your child comes out in a dramatic rash every time he eats eggs, then an allergy is clear-cut. What is less easy to sort out is the possibility of allergy related to other conditions. Some children, for instance, keep getting ear infections. Sometimes this can be the result of an allergy to cow's milk, but often it is not.

Causes

Main foods that have been implicated in childhood food allergies

Milk	Tomato
Egg	Soya
Wheat	Citrus Fruits
Cheese	Yeast
Fish	Coffee
Chocolate	

It has been shown that the type of meat least likely to cause significant reactions is lamb, the least troublesome cereal is rice, and also that peeled potatoes, lettuce, and peeled pears are also very unlikely to start any form of reaction. Some dieticians advise initial exclusion diets based primarily around just these foods, with a gradual re-introduction of other foods when all symptoms have cleared. If such a strict diet is used, a multivitamin preparation is strongly advised. You can see that such a diet is extremely strict, time-consuming, and awkward. You need to think carefully as to whether such a step is really worth it.

When to consult a doctor

If you suspect your child might be allergic to any foodstuff, it is well worth discussing the problem with your family doctor, or – if necessary- a paediatrician. If your suspicions of allergy are strong, take along a diary of symptoms and food intake. The doctor may be able to spot a link between foods that were taken before a specific symptom occurred. Alternatively he may be able to diagnose some other, nonallergic, cause for your child's symptoms. A good dietary history is perhaps the most important diagnostic test. Blood tests can sometimes help the diagnosis, but are most conclusive when there is already very strong evidence from the dietary history.

Skin tests, in which an allergen is injected into the skin and the reaction is observed, are rarely particularly specific although they can have a place. Unfortunately a positive reaction to a skin test does not necessarily prove the existence of a food allergy, and perhaps the simplest way to confirm an allergy is to withdraw that particular food from your child's diet. It sounds simple enough anyway, and so it is if your child is only allergic to shrimps, or Coca Cola. But what if you suspect a milk allergy? To exclude milk completely means carefully examining the recipes or labels for many types of bread, cake, and convenience foods. This sort of diet needs detailed advice from an expert, and your doctor should be able to put you in touch with a qualified and interested dietician. Sometimes a major exclusion, or elimination, diet must be used. In this, your child's diet will be dramatically restricted over a period of time to see if there is any change to the symptom pattern.

If excluding a suspected food leads to an apparent improvement in symptoms, that alone is not enough for the diagnosis of food allergy. It could just be coincidence. You need to give the food again to see if symptoms return, and then withdraw it to see if your child improves. If you don't apply this test you may deprive your child for years of a foodstuff that does him or her no harm at all.

How you can help

Once you have finally decided that your child has a symptom that is the result of a food allergy, then what do you do about it? Avoidance of the food is ideal, but may be difficult or simply not worthwhile. An older child may decide that a fit of sneezing is a price he is prepared to pay for a slice of chocolate cake. You should not make the treatment worse than the problem.

Treatment

If you decide that a strict diet is the answer for your child, then it is vital that nutrition is otherwise satisfactory, and so it is essential to get professional advice. Drugs such as anti-histamines may be useful if the reaction is a simple one such as an attack of hives after eating particular foods, but may be sedative and certainly aren't as good as avoiding the allergen in the first place. Another drug, disodium cromoglycate, which prevents histamine release, is promising but needs to be taken before eating the suspected food, which is not always easy.

If your child suffers from conditions such as eczema or migraine it is well worth getting more information on possible dietary triggers from your doctor or health visitor. If they cannot help, the self-help groups and other organisations listed in the appendix will almost always be able to offer advice. There is no guarantee that you will unearth a dietary cause, but it is well worth exploring the possibility.

FOOD INTOLERANCE

You may by now have noticed that I have not mentioned some of the other so-called food allergies that you have heard of elsewhere. What about gluten sensitivity, or allergy to food additives? The reason is quite simple. Though important, they are not true allergies. If you remember that an allergic reaction is a specific type of repeatable chemical reaction that always involves antibodies and allergens, all these other problems are better described as types of food intolerance. The word allergy should be reserved for true chemical allergies. Indeed this is more than just splitting hairs over definitions, as different problems require different approaches.

One of the commoner forms of food intolerance is lactose intolerance. Lactose is the natural sugar found in milk, and temporary intolerance, or inability to digest it, not uncommonly follows episodes of diarrhoea in young children. The body is unable to deal with this particular sugar, but in no way is this an allergy. While lactose intolerance is usually temporary, gluten intolerance – or coeliac disease – is far more likely to be permanent. For sufferers from this condition the presence of gluten – part of wheat, rye, barley and oats – in the bowel leads to damage to the lining of the bowel which prevents other nutrients being absorbed.

Another group of substances of which many children are intolerant are food additives. What was your immediate reaction to the phrase 'food additives'? Most people today think of additives as being entirely a bad thing, without which we would all be a lot better off. They have certainly become one of modern society's 'bad guys', being blamed for everything from behaviour disturbance in children to cancer. Indeed, if you were to read on a package that it contained additive E300 you would possibly prefer to choose something more 'natural'.

Well, E300 is vitamin C. By far the commonest food additives are sugar and salt, and there is no need to reach the automatic assumption that other chemical additives are a dreadful thing. They should all be treated in the same way as sugar and salt, in other words eaten in moderation, realising what excessive consumption can do to you.

Incidentally, not only packaged and preserved foods

contain additives. Some fresh foods such as fruit are treated with chemicals which make them look more shiny and attractive and the skins of citrus fruits occasionally have colouring added. Even meat may contain chemicals or drugs that have originally been fed to the animals to encourage growth or suppress infections.

So, do food additives do any harm? There is still no unequivocal answer, but I have little doubt that in some children certain additives do cause behavioural problems. I am equally certain that the majority of behaviour problems are not linked with food intolerance. It is much easier to blame multi-national food companies than it is to explore problems closer to home, but nevertheless I have come across very many cases where changes in the diet have helped.

Of all the behavioural problems that have been most implicated in the additive debate, hyperactivity is the most important. Hyperactive is a term that covers the child who is physically and mentally restless with boundless energy. Such children don't sit still, they talk a lot, and sleep very badly. They certainly exhaust their parents. However, the diagnosis of hyperactivity is far from definite. For example the condition is supposed to be far more common in the United States than in Britain, a difference that probably reflects doctors' attitudes rather than children's health. Some doctors even dispute that the condition exists at all, although – to quote one mother who wrote to me – 'If you doubt they exist, just try having mine for a week.'

Numerous possible causes have been examined for hyperactivity, including birth trauma, lead poisoning, petrol fumes and diet. In 1973, in California, one Dr Ben Feingold proposed that salicylates, artificial flavouring and food colouring were causes of hyperactivity. He produced two highly successful books advising diets and ways of avoiding these substances, and there did appear to be much anecdotal evidence to support his belief that a diet free of these substances helped. Since then the battle has raged, with papers regularly being published in the medical journals making claims and counter-claims. For example, one major article from the Institute of Psychiatry in London examined three reviews of the Feingold diet and concluded that any help obtained was largely a placebo response, while another report in the journal *Science* found definite impairment in the performance of learning tests when a group of hyperactive children received food colourings, although not when other 'normal' children received the colourings. The children had no idea whether they were receiving the colouring agents or not.

One of the most interesting British studies into this topic was published in 1993 and looked at a group of seventy-eight children, referred to a clinic because of hyperactive behaviour. These children were put on to a 'few foods' elimination diet, and a remarkable fifty-nine improved in behaviour during the trial. Even more remarkably, for nineteen of the children it was possible to perform a double blind trial. In other words neither the children nor their carers knew which foods were being taken. The problem foods caused impaired behaviour, and impaired psychological test performance. The authors of this academic paper concluded 'clinicians should give weight to the accounts of parents and consider this treatment in selected children with a suggestive medical history'. In particular they noted that the problem of irritability seemed to be very considerably improved.

Detailed advice on the Feingold diet, and other simpler diets, can be obtained from an organisation that has been set up for parents of hyperactive children. You will find an address in the appendix.

The final list in this section lists the food additives that the Hyperactive Children's Support Group advise should be avoided.

These are:

E102	Tartrazine	E124	Ponceau 4R
E104	Quinoline Yellow	E127	Erythrosine
E107	Yellow 2G	E128	Red 2G
E110	Sunset Yellow FCF	E132	Indigo Carmine
E120	Cochineal	E133	Brilliant Blue FCF
E122	Carmoisine	E211	Sodium benzoate
E123	Amaranth	E220	Sulphur dioxide
E150	Caramel	E250	Sodium nitrate
E15I	Black PN	E251	Potassium nitrite
E154	Brown FK	E320	Butylated hydroxyamisole
E155	Brown H		
E210	Benzoic Acid	E321	Butylated hydroxytoluene

Although the debate is likely to continue for some time yet, I think all the evidence suggests that a small but significant group of children with behaviour problems are genuinely affected adversely by food additives. As a result it is well worth trying such a diet, but the process is not easy, requires constant supervision, and carries the considerable danger that if it fails, parents may feel it is just because they are not trying hard enough and may put their child on stricter and stricter diets. Do not fall into this trap. If dietary change does not solve your child's behavioural or hyperactivity problem, then look for other causes and ways of helping. Do not let it become an obsession.

THE LUNGS

The problem of allergy causing wheezing is dealt with very

fully in the chapter on 'The child who wheezes'. The basic underlying problem is again just the same as in the eyes or nose. The tubes in the lungs, known as the bronchi, are lined with mast cells. They also have a layer of muscle. Release of histamine from the mast cells will cause an asthma attack to develop, with the muscles tightening and the tubes narrowing. This particularly affects the smaller tubes in the lung (the larger tubes being held open by rings of cartilage) and as a result it becomes much harder to breathe out than to breathe in. Because of the tightness in the tubes, you can hear the typical wheeze as air flows in and out.

As well as the obstruction to air flow in the bronchi, the very smallest tubes in the lungs may shut down almost completely. This leads to a fall in the amount of oxygen that is able to get into the body, and as a result the patient becomes breathless.

The principles of treatment are the same as for allergic rhinitis, in particular involving inhaled anti-inflammatory drugs (typically steroids), inhaled disodium cromoglycate (Intal), and a number of other drugs that are dealt with in full in the section of this book on 'Asthma' (page 52).

ANAPHYLACTIC SHOCK

If an antigen is able to get directly into the blood stream, for instance if a child is bitten by an insect to which he or she is allergic, then the allergic reaction that I described earlier in this section can happen almost everywhere in the body all at once. Mast cells all over the body can be affected, and there is a sudden outpouring of enormous quantities of histamine. This causes the serious condition known as anaphylactic shock. This can also occur with antigens that are taken in by mouth in people who are particularly susceptible to these. Certain food, including eggs, fish, cow's milk protein, and nuts (particularly peanuts), are well known to produce anaphylaxis in susceptible individuals. Children who are allergic to nuts have to be particularly careful as nut products can turn up in all sorts of unexpected food-stuffs. For instance, many biscuits contain peanuts, and some food labels say 'vegetable oil' when they should say they contain 'arachis oil' – the alternative name for peanut oil. Up to forty per cent of children affected by nut allergy will have their first reaction before the age of two. It is interesting to note that even some nipple creams contain nut oil, which could be where babies get their first exposure and sensitisation. The parents of children with severe food allergies need to become expert in reading food labels.

The symptoms are dramatic and unmistakable. Within a very short time – possibly in less than a minute – weals appear all over the body. The skin on the face becomes very swollen, and the eyelids may swell so much that they close. The lips, too, may swell dramatically, as may the tongue and the lining of the mouth. If the sufferer also suffers from asthma, severe wheezing may occur. Because of the amount of fluid that is poured out into all the weals across the body, the blood pressure may drop, making the heart race and the sufferer feel faint.

The treatment for this condition is an immediate injection of adrenaline. Ring both 999 and call a doctor for this immediately. The doctor may also need to give other drugs such as steroids, but adrenaline is the life-saver.

Whilst you are waiting, if your child is able to swallow, and you can give him or her a dose of anti-histamine this may help slightly, but by itself it won't be enough. Otherwise it is important to stay with your child, trying your very hardest to keep him or her calm. Fear and panic greatly worsen the situation. If by any chance your child stops breathing, perform C.P.R. (cardio-pulmonary resuscitation) immediately. See page 330 for details.

If you or your child are seriously allergic to anything, then your doctor may provide you with adrenaline and a needle and syringe to give this, along with full instructions as to what to do. Alternatively some doctors may provide automatic syringes that are significantly easier to use. The sort of patient who is ideally suited to having adrenaline readily available is someone who may be allergic to bee stings and lives in a village where there is a bee hive.

The child with red eyes

Symptoms

The number one symptom suffered by a child with red eyes is, hardly surprisingly, red eyes! However there are a number of important different causes of red eyes, and a number of associated symptoms, such as soreness, grittiness, blurring of vision, or headache, which can also help to unravel the likely cause.

Unusual redness – of almost any part of the body – is usually a sign of inflammation, and red eyes are caused by inflammation of different parts of the eye. To understand this, a brief description of the normal eye anatomy is necessary.

The simplest way to understand the anatomy of the eye is to follow the path taken by light as it enters the eye and subsequently strikes the retina at the back of the eye. First of all, the light passes through the thin transparent cornea across the front of the eye, before it reaches the lens itself. Between the cornea and the lens there is a space filled with a watery liquid known as the aqueous humor. Stretched across the whole of the front of the white of the eye, and also lining the eyelids, is a membrane called the conjunctiva.

The iris, the part of the eye that gives it colour, is in the aqueous humor between the cornea and the lens. The dark spot in the centre of the eye is the pupil, and this lies in the centre of the iris. The pupil changes size depending on how much light falls upon it. In dark conditions, the eye needs

Horizontal Cross Section of the Eye

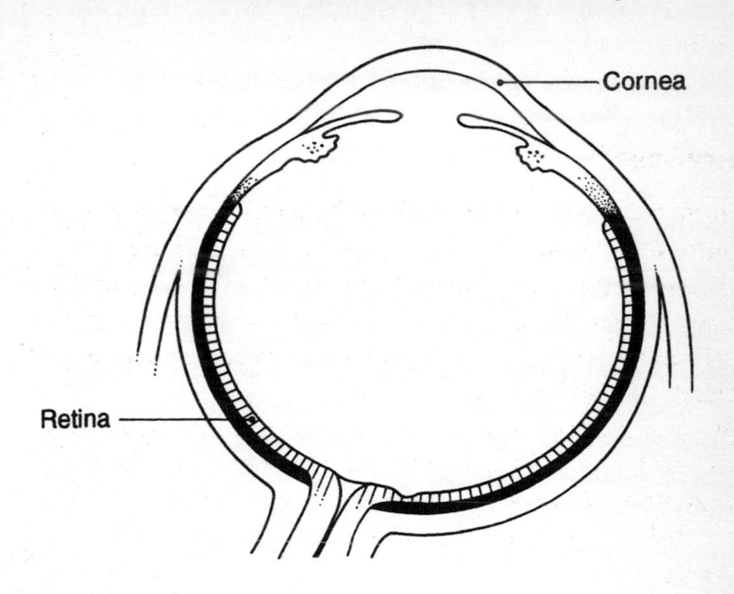

Detail of the Front of the Eye

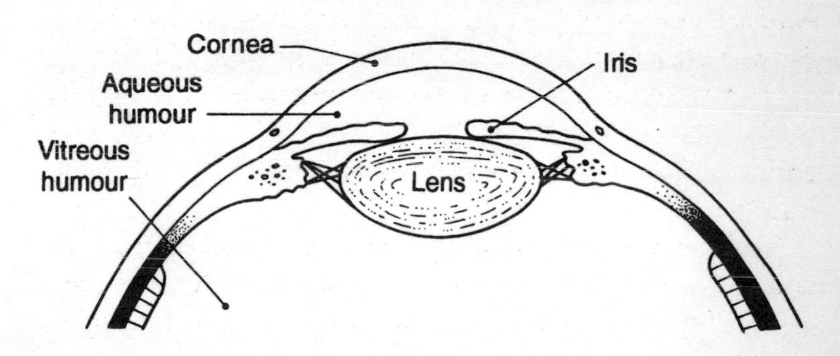

more light to be able to see clearly, and the pupil therefore opens wide to allow more light in. In very bright conditions, the amount of light needs to be restricted, so the pupil shuts down to a much smaller size.

The lens focuses the beam of light through another clear fluid-filled chamber, the vitreous humor, onto the retina. The retina is the equivalent of a film in a camera, and it converts the light impulses into nervous signals which are transmitted to the visual part of the brain along the optic nerve.

In addition to the eye itself, the eyelids keep the front of the eye clean, and free from particles of dust and other irritants. Tears are produced as a highly effective antiseptic which also keeps the eye clean and free from infection.

Almost every part of the eye can be subject to inflammation, and if the inflammation affects a part that is visible the net result is a red eye.

Causes

By far the commonest cause of a red eye is conjunctivitis. This is the word that describes inflammation of the conjunctivae. Such inflammation can be caused by infection, or by allergy. Other causes of a red eye are extremely rare in children, but are important and are dealt with briefly later in this chapter.

The eye can also appear red if it has suffered some form of direct irritation. A common cause is the chlorine that is added to the water of swimming pools. Many children finish a session of swimming with two red sore eyes, but this soon passes after the effect of the chlorine wears off – either helped by being washed out with a shower, or with tears. A single red eye can be caused by local irritation to that eye from, for instance, an eyelash that has turned in, a particle of dust, a scratch, or even a tiny insect.

Sticky eyes, with or without redness, are very common indeed in newborn babies. Sticky yellow or cream-coloured pus may build up overnight and the eyelids may even be stuck together in the morning. Gentle wiping with cotton wool dipped in warm water may be all that is needed. When you do this, wipe from the inside corner of the eye outwards. In such newborn sticky eyes, antibiotic drops are rarely essential, except when the whites of the eyes also become red or inflamed.

If the eyelids, rather than the conjunctivae, become inflamed or infected, the condition is known as blepharitis. Less common in a child is inflammation of the iris, or iritis (discussed later in this section).

The symptoms of conjunctivitis largely depend on the cause. In all forms of conjunctivitis there will be redness of the conjunctivae. This is mainly seen in the whites of the eye and the lining of the eyelids. If the cause is infection there is also likely to be discharge, particularly in the mornings, and a sensation of stickiness and grittiness of the eyes.

In allergic conjunctivitis there tends to be itchiness and redness, but without the stickiness or gritty sensation. Allergic conjunctivitis is frequently a symptom of hayfever, or perennial rhinitis (the year-round version of hayfever), and may be associated with a runny or blocked nose. Children with such allergies also are frequently sufferers from either eczema or asthma, or may come from families where these problems are common.

Sometimes you may see a separate area of very bright red colour in the white of your child's eye. This is almost certainly a sub-conjunctival haemorrhage – which sounds much worse than it really is. It is actually a spontaneous bursting of a tiny blood vessel in the conjunctiva that is usually triggered by something that causes a sudden rise in pressure – such as coughing, sneezing, screaming, being knocked on the eye, or even intense straining if the child is very constipated. These haemorrhages are entirely harmless and will fade over the next few weeks, leaving no damage whatsoever.

One final condition that can cause a red eye is iritis. This causes slightly different symptoms. The redness tends to be at its maximum near the iris, and the pupil is likely to be smaller in the affected eye than in the normal eye. The condition may also cause pain in the eye or blurring of vision, and any or all of these symptoms are a reason to see your doctor the same day. Iritis is actually quite rare in children, but it can be easily treated if seen promptly – and can lead to permanent problems with vision if treatment is delayed.

When to consult a doctor

Unless the cause of conjunctivitis is very obvious – for instance redness that comes on immediately following a swim in a swimming pool – then you should take your child to be assessed by the doctor. If you think your child may have a foreign body in the eye, then you can try washing this out with water, or gently lifting the eyelid and trying to remove the foreign body with a piece of cotton wool. However if this does not work then seek professional help. If there is any possibility of a fragment of metal having gone in the eye, then it is best to take your child to a local hospital casualty where the eye can be X-rayed, but non-metallic foreign bodies can usually be sorted out by your local practice.

You should very definitely consult a doctor right away if:

- Your child has a single red eye that isn't sticky. The cause may be a condition such as uveitis (inflammation of the uvea, which consists of the iris, the ciliary body, and the choroid) or iritis and this needs medical treatment.

- Your child develops a red eye after any form of poke in the eye or other eye injury. It is possible that the surface of the cornea may have been scratched. The doctor will be able to detect this using a special staining eye drop known as fluorescein, and treatment using antibiotic drops or possibly ointment is important to avoid scarring which might later affect eyesight.
- Your child complains that his or her eyesight is in any way abnormal. Conjunctivitis does not affect the eyesight, apart from a slight blurring that is usually cured by blinking or wiping away the matter in the eye.
- Your child has a foreign body in the eye that you cannot get out easily.
- There is any possibility that a foreign body may have penetrated the eyeball. If the child has been watching someone grinding or chiselling at metal or stone and a piece flew into the eye at speed, this can break through the surface of the eyeball and does need dealing with urgently.

How you can help

Infectious conjunctivitis can spread very easily around families, schools, or playgroups. It is highly contagious, and therefore scrupulous hygiene is essential. You should always use a separate flannel and towel for the affected child, and wash your hands carefully after using the eye drops or ointment. Children with infectious conjunctivitis should always be kept off school, playgroup, or other communal activities until the condition is completely clear.

As well as using any treatment prescribed by your doctor,

you can gently wipe the eyes clean using cotton wool soaked in clean warm water. This is particularly soothing if there has been a build-up of discharge overnight.

Treatment

Infectious conjunctivitis

Conjunctivitis is usually treated by using antibiotic drops or ointment. Children are often frightened of this procedure, so if your child is old enough try to explain what you are doing first, and try to avoid any sudden movements that will make your child jerk away from you. You may need help in putting drops or ointment into a young child's eyes. It is easiest if the child looks upwards, and you put your thumb on the skin of the cheek just under the eye. Gentle downward pressure rolls the eyelid slightly open and it is then relatively easy to insert the drops or ointment. Ointment is usually best put just inside the lower eyelid. When your child closes his or her eye, the ointment will be spread over the surface of the eye. This will feel a bit sticky for a short while but this will soon pass off.

Without treatment, infectious conjunctivitis is likely to persist for anything up to three weeks, but it will be cleared rapidly with antibiotic drops or ointments. These should usually be used until the condition is better, and then for another twenty-four hours.

This condition is very common indeed in the first eighteen months of life, and your child may have very frequent attacks. This is not a cause for alarm or concern, and the condition almost always rights itself. However if it persists after eighteen months, then your G.P. is likely to refer your child to a local ophthalmologist as the most likely cause will be a blocked tear duct.

The tear ducts are situated at the inner corner of each lower eyelid, and they allow drainage of tears – which are being produced all the time – into the nose. A blockage leads to a constant apparent slight watering of the eyes, and frequently infection will set in. Very frequently the problem resolves spontaneously in the first year and a half of life, and you may be able to help it clear by gentle massaging of the lower eyelid near the nose. However if nature does not sort it out, the problem can be easily remedied by a gentle probing by the ophthalmologist to clear the ducts.

Allergic conjunctivitis

If the allergic conjunctivitis is part of a wider picture of allergy, perhaps being associated with nasal symptoms, then it may be most effectively treated with oral anti-histamines. The older anti-histamines such as chlorpheniramine (Piriton) were fairly sedative, but modern drugs such as terfenadine (Triludan) should not make your child sleepy.

If either anti-histamines alone are not enough, or you or your doctor prefer using a topical treatment (one that is used on the surface rather than being taken internally) then your child may be prescribed eye drops such as disodium cromoglycate (Opticrom). These are remarkably free of side effects, but have to be used four times a day every day.

Prevention

If you can identify the cause of any conjunctivitis, then you may be able to avoid this in future. A child with allergic conjunctivitis triggered by cigarette smoke, for instance, would be much better off if you didn't smoke, and your house was a no-smoking zone. However such avoidance is not always possible.

Conjunctivitis that is caused by infection is generally very infectious indeed, and you can prevent spread to others if you follow the advice scrupulously on hygiene that I have described above.

The child with other eye problems

Whilst the previous section dealt with the child with red eyes, this brief section looks at four other eye problems:

The child with a squint
The child with a cloudy eye
The child with a stye
The child with swollen eyelids

THE CHILD WITH A SQUINT

Both eyes should look in exactly the same direction. They should be perfectly parallel. Squinting is the term used when the eyes are looking in different directions. Whilst it is not uncommon for children to have an occasional squint in the first couple of months of life (but *not* a persistent squint), after this age squints always need medical attention.

Understanding and acting on this really is vital. Normally, both eyes work in parallel, and whilst the brain receives two separate sets of signals from the two eyes, it combines these together into a single stereoscopic image. If the eyes are not perfectly in synch with each other, the brain cannot produce a single image and the child sees double. If you have ever seen double (should you ever have overindulged in alcohol for instance) you will know what a disconcerting experience this can be. However, in small children it is far more than just disconcerting. The brain copes with the double image by suppressing the weaker one altogether. A squint that goes untreated in the long-term will result in a loss of vision in one of the eyes. I have at least one adult patient who is blind in one eye simply because a squint was ignored when she was a child.

This is the reason that doctors seem so concerned about picking up squints. I know that I occasionally puzzle parents when they have brought their child in with a sore throat, and I, suspecting that I have glimpsed a squint, suddenly start checking their child's eyes, but with possible squints it really is essential to be certain.

If your doctor confirms the presence of a squint, he or she will arrange for a full assessment by a hospital orthoptic or ophthalmology department. There are many possible causes for squints, although the commonest is an imbalance in the muscles that control eye movements. In older children the cause might be a problem such as long-sightedness which leads to excessive accommodation (the focus adjustment of the eye) and which can lead to the eye turning inwards.

Sometimes, what appears to be a squint in a young child is actually an optical illusion caused by the relative broadness of the nose at that age, but even if you aren't sure whether your child has a squint or not, please don't take any risks.

THE CHILD WITH A CLOUDY EYE

The fluid in the eye should always appear clear. This is the fluid that you can see through the centre of the pupil. If the pupil or iris appear in any way cloudy, then it is essential that you consult your doctor right away. A cloudy appearance is never normal, and the conditions that can cause it, whilst rare, all need immediate medical attention.

In adults the two commonest causes of such cloudiness are cataract (a thickening of the lens), and glaucoma (an increase in pressure in the fluid inside the eyeball).

Whilst these are both very rare in children, they are by no means impossible, and can even appear as congenital conditions.

THE CHILD WITH A STYE

A stye is a small abscess, or boil, in or near the hair follicles of the eyelashes. They are typically red swellings, often the size of a pea, on the edge of the eyelid, though they may begin with general redness and a slight swelling of the lid before the actual lump appears.

Styes hurt, and are much more comfortable when they have burst. However, please do not attempt to squeeze them. Warm compresses (cotton wool that has been soaked in warm – but not too hot!) water, can certainly help to bring them to a head. Steam also helps. A good old-fashioned, but effective treatment is to wrap the large end of a wooden spoon in a piece of cloth, dip this in very hot water, and hold this near to the stye. However, you must make sure that the hot material does not touch the skin, and that the hot water cannot be spilt.

The great majority of styes will burst and heal without needing any further medical attention. If a stye persists without pointing, or coming to a head, for more than two or three days, do consult your doctor. In addition, if they keep occurring then an antibiotic ointment from the doctor may eradicate any bacteria that are being carried and can help to prevent recurrences. Incidentally, whilst any member of your family has a stye, he or she should use a separate flannel and towel to prevent spreading.

THE CHILD WITH SWOLLEN EYELIDS

The tissues around the eyes are very soft and sensitive. They can swell up after relatively trivial irritation or injury. Whilst sometimes the cause of swollen eyelids is unimportant, on other occasions it is the sign of something serious. This brief section should help you to distinguish between the two. Obviously, if you know the cause – an insect bite or an injury, for instance – then these diagnostic aids do not apply. In general, if a condition affects only one eye then the cause will be local to that eye – such as infection or injury. Where both eyes are affected, then the cause will be general – such as an allergy or fluid retention.

Conditions affecting both eyes

Both eyelids are swollen and associated with itching and watering:

This can be caused by allergic conjunctivitis. See page 267.

Both eyelids are swollen and puffy, with no itching or redness:

This can be caused by fluid retention, and one possible cause of this is a condition called nephrotic syndrome, in which the kidneys leak protein into the urine. Nephrotic syndrome also tends to be associated with puffiness of the ankles, feet, and hands. If this appears to be happening, consult your doctor and ideally take a specimen of your child's urine with you as your doctor will want to test this for the presence or absence of protein.

Conditions affecting only one eye

One eyelid is red and swollen, but with no fever:

This may be the beginning of a stye.

One eyelid is red and swollen, and the child has a fever:

This could be one of two potentially serious infections:

periorbital cellulitis (an infection of the tissues in front of the eye) or orbital cellulitis (an infection of the eye socket). Both of these need urgent medical attention.

The child who has a fit

Fits (or convulsions – they are the same thing) can be truly terrifying. Most parents feel totally helpless when faced with their child having a convulsion, especially if it is for the first time. What can be even more confusing is trying to unravel whether your child has actually had a convulsion, or a faint (see page 281), or even just the tremors that come with a high temperature. This chapter will explain the various different types of convulsion, explain what the causes are, and give you advice on how to handle the situation. Incidentally, it is important to realise that not every child who has a fit is necessarily epileptic. Although there is no difference between an 'ordinary fit' and an 'epileptic fit', a child is only described as epileptic if he or she has repeated fits where no obvious trigger is noted.

WHAT IS A CONVULSION?

Convulsions are typically caused by a burst of abnormal activity in the brain. The brain normally functions like a computer with billions of electrical impulses being passed between cells controlling all our bodily functions. Normally all this electrical activity is highly controlled, but in a convulsion the messages become completely scrambled, and this uninhibited over-activity of the brain cells temporarily interrupts the normal way that the brain functions. Convulsions can be of two main types – *generalised*, which involves the whole of the brain, and *focal* which affects only part of the brain.

In children there are two main types of convulsion, known as 'tonic-clonic seizures' (these used to be called 'grand mal') and 'absence seizures' (which used to be called 'petit mal'). In a tonic-clonic seizure the child goes unconscious, goes stiff, falls over, and then the limbs may shake uncontrollably. It is the most common type of fit, and may well also be associated with tongue biting, incontinence, and is followed by a period of drowsiness – and probably amnesia for what has happened.

In absence seizures, the child suddenly stops what he or she is doing, looks vacant, appears to stare momentarily, and then carries on with what he or she was doing. These may occur without anyone noticing at all, or even just thinking the child is day-dreaming.

However there are over forty different types of seizure, and everyone who experiences fits is affected in a different way. The British Epilepsy Association produce a couple of excellent booklets – 'Epilepsy and Everyone' and 'Epilepsy and Children' – and I recommend these to you if you want to understand the subject. Their address is in the appendix.

There are two sorts of fit which are by far the commonest in children, febrile and epileptic:

FEBRILE CONVULSIONS

By far the commonest of these are febrile convulsions. These typically occur between the ages of six months and five years – with a majority being in the second year – and are associated with, and also triggered by, a sudden rise in temperature. Approximately four per cent of children will experience at least one of these convulsions, and there may well be a history of convulsions in the family.

Causes

The fit can be triggered by anything that causes a raised temperature – such as an ear infection, urine infection, or sore throat. If any of us were put in a high enough temperature it is likely we would have a fit, simply because of the disruption to the brain. In febrile convulsions the child's brain appears to be more sensitive than usual to these changes in temperature, and this triggers a discharge of electrical activity which leads to a full-blown generalised convulsion which can last for several minutes. The symptoms of a febrile convulsion may well be exactly the same as the symptoms of any other form of convulsion: the child loses consciousness and his or her arms and legs twitch uncontrollably for a few minutes. Typically, the child will be drowsy after regaining consciousness.

When to consult a doctor

If your child has a first febrile convulsion, call the doctor. It is absolutely essential that the first fit in any child is thoroughly assessed to ensure that this is truly the diagnosis. It is likely that he or she will be admitted to hospital for assessment, although this is less usual for subsequent convulsions.

How you can help

- If it is a first convulsion, call the doctor
- Lie your child on the floor, away from any hard objects or sharp objects
- Lie your child on the side so that saliva or mucus can drain out of the mouth rather than being inhaled
- Make sure that you cool your child down. If you can, strip

him or her down, and even use tepid sponging to lower the temperature. Do not lie your child in front of a raging fire. This is a great recipe for keeping the convulsion going

- Do not put anything in the child's mouth for him or her to bite on. This may damage a tooth, and do more harm than good
- If this is not a first convulsion and it lasts for more than ten minutes call a doctor or ambulance
- Once the emergency is over, discuss with your doctor the possibility of you having a supply of an anti-convulsant which you could administer on future occasions

Treatment

If the convulsion has lasted more than fifteen minutes, the doctor is likely to give an anti-convulsant drug. The most commonly used drug is diazepam, and this is typically given into the rectum, using a special applicator.

Prevention

To prevent future convulsions, always try to act promptly if your child seems to be developing a raised temperature. This involves using paracetamol, stripping off excess clothing, and even using tepid sponging. If febrile convulsions keep happening despite your using all these measures, your child may need preventative medication to stop further attacks. It is highly likely that your child will grow out of the problem completely by the age of six. Only about one child in fifty who has febrile convulsions will go on to have epilepsy. In addition, a recent study of 300 children who had febrile convulsions showed that at the age of fourteen years their I.Q. and intellectual performance was every bit as good as children who had never had a fit.

EPILEPSY

In the United Kingdom, one person in every 130 has epilepsy, so it is far from being a real rarity. It is a brain disorder which results in spontaneous disordered electrical activity, but – despite what some people believe – the great majority of children with epilepsy have absolutely normal intelligence.

Symptoms

The epileptic attacks may take any of the forms described on page 274.

As well as the tonic-clonic seizure and absence seizures described above, there are also 'sleep seizures' which only affect the child when he or she is asleep, and so which may obviously be missed as no one witnesses them. Sometimes the only clue might be a bitten tongue, or some other associated symptom. In infancy there is also a condition known as 'infantile spasms' which may occur several times in a day. These occur suddenly, with short sharp episodes where the child curls up and then flexes the whole body, and then relaxes, sometimes with a short sharp cry. This is a rare condition, but potentially extremely serious and it is essential that it is diagnosed and treated as soon as possible.

When to consult a doctor

After the first time that your child has one of these attacks he or she will always be referred to hospital for thorough investigation. This will include a test known as an electro-encephalogram (E.E.G.) which measures the electrical activity of the brain and can pinpoint what form of convulsion is occurring, and why these may be occurring.

How you can help

The British Epilepsy Association makes a number of important recommendations about helping your child with epilepsy. Some of these are as follows:

- Accept your child for what he is – a unique individual who happens to have convulsions – and encourage him to do the same
- Make sure each of your children has a fair share of your time, interest, and energy
- Concentrate on what he or she can do, rather than what he or she can't
- Have fun together as a family
- Don't rush in to help, unless your child obviously needs it
- Don't restrict your family life because of the epilepsy
- Don't treat your child with epilepsy differently from others
- Don't allow your child to think of himself as 'sick' or use epilepsy as an excuse

The British Epilepsy Association's advice is so very sensible, and so very positive, that I really would urge every parent of a child with epilepsy to contact them and take advantage of their positive, authoritative common sense.

Treatment

If your child does turn out to have epilepsy, he or she will need to start treatment with medication which is designed to be taken regularly in order to prevent the convulsions. If you can identify anything that triggers a convulsion – sitting close to the television, for instance – then this too should be avoided. The whole aim of treatment is to give your child as normal and active a life as is humanly possible. The vast majority of children with epilepsy live totally normal, happy lives.

Medication will normally be continued until your child has been fit-free for at least two years. You really do need to take a positive outlook so that your child has as normal and happy a childhood as possible.

Prevention

In the initial stages of epilepsy, until your child's convulsions have been brought under control, there are some activities that it would be wise to avoid, activities where a sudden fit could be dangerous. These include cycling in traffic, or swimming alone – though swimming with a responsible adult is obviously fine.

COPING WITH A CONVULSION

It is obviously essential that you should know how to cope with a child that is having a convulsion. The guidelines are quite straightforward:

- Lie your child on the floor on his or her side, so that if he dribbles or vomits this can drain out of the mouth and not be inhaled.
- Do not put anything in your child's mouth. The old idea about putting a spoon handle into the mouth to stop tongue biting is positively dangerous and can damage the teeth (not to mention the spoon!). In any case, when tongue biting occurs it happens at the beginning of the fit, so that by the time you can do anything to prevent it, you are too late.
- Do not try to get hold of your child's tongue. You will get bitten.

- Simply wait for the convulsion to end. If it seems to be a prolonged fit, or is different from other fits that your child has experienced, then call your doctor. If your child regularly has fits then discuss with your doctor about when he or she should be notified, and when you can simply let the convulsion run its course.
- Check for breathing after the fit has come to an end, but never start resuscitation (such as C.P.R. – cardio-pulmonary resuscitation – or the 'kiss of life') whilst your child is still convulsing. Many children are a little blue after a convulsion, but usually breathing rapidly returns their colour to normal.
- If your child has a high temperature, try to cool him or her down, by stripping off clothing, gentle fanning, or even tepid sponging. Do not try to give paracetamol by mouth whilst the convulsion is still going on.

FAINTS

Causes

Faints are quite different from fits, although it can occasionally require quite detailed tests to discriminate one from the other. Fainting is caused by a sudden drop of blood pressure, and may appear completely out of the blue, although it is more likely to be associated with a raised temperature, exertion, a hot room, upset or shock, or suddenly standing up from a sitting or crouching position. The fall in blood pressure means that insufficient blood reaches the brain, and fainting is nature's way of making you lie down – which brings the head to the same level as the heart and allows blood to reach the brain again.

Symptoms

Typically the child will know that the faint is going to happen. He or she feels hot and sweaty, may complain of a curious buzzing sound in the ears, and of black spots appearing in their vision. The child may appear to be sweaty and pale before he or she collapses and becomes unconscious. Recovery will be complete after a minute or two at the most. There is never any tongue biting or incontinence, and if the child is able to sit down or lower the head between the knees, it is possible to stop the faint coming on at all. However, if your child has repeated episodes of fainting, your doctor may want to arrange investigations to make quite certain that these are not a type of convulsion, however unusual this may be.

The child with bone or joint problems

Entire books have been written about single joints, so this chapter can only begin to look at the more important conditions that can cause problems for children and their parents. I shall initially look at injuries, then briefly consider each of the major joints in turn.

Fractures and other injuries

This morning in surgery I saw a five-year-old boy who might as well have a season ticket to our local casualty unit. He seems to make a habit of falling, twisting, banging and bruising himself, and has had more X-rays already than most of us have in a lifetime. He is not unusual. Many is the happy afternoon I have spent in casualty units with my son, particularly after he took up rugger at school. Whilst most serious injuries are likely to end up at an accident and emergency department, parents do need to understand how best they can help.

After even a minor injury, your child is likely to be reluctant to use the affected part for a short while. However, after most bruises and sprains most children are soon ready to get back into action, and, having seemed to be mortally injured one minute, are off running with their friends the next.

None the less, fractures are not uncommon in children. As their bones are still growing, a relatively minor break can disrupt the way that the bone grows, and so should be taken seriously. If a child is reluctant to move an arm or leg after he or she injures it, then you should be highly suspicious that there may be a fracture, and should seek medical advice right away. However, even for the most skilled of doctors, it can be extraordinarily difficult to tell if a bone is fractured without taking an X-ray. Sprains can cause as much swelling as fractures, if not more, and some minor fractures may not show up on the initial X-rays. Small children are particularly prone to an injury known as a green-stick fracture. If you try to snap a piece of twig that is still alive and green, it does not crack right through, but instead one side cracks slightly whilst the other just flexes. This is exactly what can happen in a fracture in childhood.

The main signs of a fracture are:

- Swelling over a bone
- Tenderness that is isolated to one small area of bone
- A child who is reluctant to use that arm or leg
- Pain or swelling that lasts for more than a day or so

If in doubt, seek help. The bone may well not be fractured, but it is usually important that you should know.

THE LEGS

Bow legs

All children appear to be bow-legged up to the age of two, and have legs that look as if they have spent a lifetime riding horses. This is the result of the moulding of the bones that takes place whilst the child is still in the womb. In the enormous majority of children the legs gradually straighten out, but in some – in particular children who are overweight – the bowing may last almost up to the age of four. If your child seems to be getting more bow-legged in his or her fourth year, seek medical advice, though very few children need surgical correction of the bowing. Only in exceptional cases will there be a need for special exercises, braces, or shoes to encourage bowing to straighten out.

Also seek medical advice if the bowing only seems to affect one leg.

Knock knees

These are also entirely normal in children at the age of three or four. It is as if the legs start bowed, then go too far in the other direction, and only end up straight some time around the age of ten. It is very rare for treatment to be needed for this condition. Special shoes and wedges occasionally help, and you should only need medical help if one leg is much worse than the other, or if your child seems unusually knock-kneed compared to other children of the same age.

Painful legs

Many children, particularly between the ages of four and eight, complain of a vague aching in the legs. This is often worse in the evening, and tends not to be a problem during the day. It is usually felt deep in the thigh or the lower leg. Such pains can even wake a child from his or her sleep, and have been described for years as 'growing pains'. I find this an entirely unconvincing explanation for the pain, but have not seen any really good explanation for what causes such pains. Growing pains never ever make a child limp, or complain of pain localised to a joint, so if your child has either of these conditions seek medical advice right away. In addition, it would be wise to seek help if the pain only ever happens in one leg.

The best treatment for these pains is paracetamol or

ibuprofen, gentle massage, a warm hot water bottle, and cuddles and reassurance when appropriate.

Painful knees

Painful knees are not common in small children, and if they occur you should seek medical advice. However in children aged ten years or more, pain can result from a not-uncommon condition called Osgood-Schlatter's disease. In these children there is a swollen and tender lump towards the top of the front of the tibia. This is caused by inflammation at the point where the tendon that holds the kneecap joins the upper tibia, and is much more common in athletic children who enjoy games and sports. As traditionally the main treatment has been avoiding games and sports, this seems more than a little unfair. The condition is not serious, usually subsides as growing ceases, but you should still seek your doctor's assessment and advice.

Noisy knees

Knees that are noisy, but not painful, that clunk and click, but which don't interfere with running or playing or climbing, are harmless. If the knee locks, or gives way, or causes your child any upset other than being noisy, then get it examined by a doctor.

Limping

Simple things can obviously make a child limp. Problems with footwear, a painful verruca, infected eczema affecting the foot, a recent injection on that side – all these are possible minor causes. However, if a child limps and there is no very clearly discernible reason for the limp, then it is essential you have your child assessed by a doctor.

A common cause of limping in small children can be an irritable hip. This may follow a virus infection, and is caused by an inflammation of the synovium, or lining of the hip joint. It usually recovers after rest, but your doctor may very well want to arrange an urgent X-ray to make sure that the hip is otherwise normal.

Less common, but more important, is Perthes' disease. This typically occurs in children aged between four and ten years, and usually affects only one hip. The initial symptom is limping, and the child then complains of slight pain which may be felt either in the hip or the knee (even though the problem is in the hip).

In Perthes' disease, the blood supply to the growing part of the upper thigh-bone (the femur) becomes reduced, and the bone becomes softened and inflamed. The diseased part of the bone actually dies, and as the femur grows this damaged bone will be replaced by new bone. The aim of treatment is to protect this newly growing bone.

For this reason, any child between the ages of four and ten who limps for more than twenty-four hours should see a doctor who will arrange for him or her to see an orthopaedic specialist. With correct treatment, the outlook for this condition is good.

Limping may also be associated with conditions such as osteomyelitis (see page 294) and Lyme disease (page 215).

Hip problems

All newborn babies are assessed almost immediately after birth to check for congenital dislocation of the hip (C.D.H.) This affects seven out of every 1,000 children, girls more than boys, and there may well be a family history of the condition. The hip joint is a ball and socket joint, and if the ball and socket do not fit together correctly – for instance if the socket is too shallow – the ball can slide out of the socket. Early detection of this problem can prevent long-term problems with the hip joint and with walking, and treatment usually involves splinting of the joint to hold the hip joint in its socket as it grows.

C.D.H. is usually tested for by manipulating the newborn baby's thighs which can sometimes be made to click. By no means do all 'clicky hips' turn out to have C.D.H., but it is at least a sign that more investigation is required.

If, whilst changing your baby's nappy, you notice a click or a clunk as you move the thighs, particularly whilst opening them out, then this may be a sign of a problem with the hip joint – though could equally just be a twanging sensation from a tendon. Ask your doctor or health visitor to check it out when you next see them.

THE FEET

Pigeon toes

Pigeon toes, or intoeing, can be caused by a number of possible factors, but the great majority of children grow out of the condition. Sometimes there is inward rotation of the upper part of the femur (the thigh-bone), sometimes there is inward twisting of the lower shin-bone, and sometimes the foot is simply curved inwards at the level of the toes. I shall look at each of these briefly at the end of this section.

Normally the condition will have resulted from the rather cramped conditions inside the mother's uterus, and it should be possible gently to manoeuvre the foot and toes into a more normal-looking shape. If they simply won't move, and the foot seems to be fixed in an abnormal position, then this may be a form of club foot, and you should seek medical advice, although this will normally have been noticed at birth.

Small children who are learning to walk appear to try and grip the ground with their toes. This can create an illusion of pigeon toeing. As they develop more confidence in walking, the feet will appear more normal.

Do not waste your money on special shoes that are supposed to correct pigeon toeing. As the condition usually recovers spontaneously, these are entirely unnecessary.

If the pigeon toeing is bad enough to make your child trip up when he or she walks, if it persists past the age of ten, or if it only affects one side, then you should seek medical advice.

As discussed above, pigeon toes can have several causes:

Inward rotation of the upper part of the femur

If the upper thigh is twisted inwards, then the whole leg will be twisted with it, and this makes the feet appear pigeon-toed. You can encourage your child to sit cross-legged on the floor, as this encourages the femur to rotate outwards. In ninety-nine per cent of children this condition will correct itself spontaneously, and doctors only really need to treat very severe cases or those that persist well after the age of ten.

Inward twisting of the lower shin-bone

This condition is known as tibial torsion, and the vast majority of cases recover spontaneously and need no treatment and no exercise. However, if it is severe, your doctor may refer you to a paediatric orthopaedic surgeon for an assessment. Occasionally a night splint may be used to correct the angulation.

Curved feet

Many babies are born with a curve to the inner border of the feet. This is almost certainly a result of the way the baby was lying in the uterus, and the enormous majority of these will have cleared up spontaneously by one year of age. If the curve is really bad, or does not recover spontaneously, then you should certainly seek medical advice, but this will usually be spotted by your health visitor during regular checks.

Flat feet

Doctors used to worry a great deal about flat feet, until someone noticed that the first three people to run a four-minute mile had apparently all had flat feet! Flat feet by themselves do not matter. They should only be a cause for concern if they cause any pain on walking. Many small children appear to have flat feet because the normal arch of the foot is filled in by fat and other tissues. Typically, by the age of five years this fat will have disappeared and the normal arch of the foot will have become visible.

If your child still appears to have flat feet after the age of five, ask him or her to stand on tiptoe. Normally, when a child does this the normal arch of the foot appears. If no arch does appear, then further assessment may be necessary. In addition, any form of flat foot that is painful should be assessed too.

In the child who does develop an arch on tiptoe, then there is no underlying problem, and the only problem this type of flat foot can cause is uneven wearing of the shoes. Insoles or wedges can help, but do talk to a doctor about this first. He or she may make a referral to a physiotherapist or chiropodist.

Walking on the toes

Very many children walk on their toes when they first learn to walk, particularly under the age of one year. If your child continues to walk on his or her toes after this, then check that he or she is able to stand with the feet flat on the ground. If this is possible, then it is most unlikely that there is a problem and the condition should resolve spontaneously. If your child cannot stand comfortably with both heels on the ground, then the problem might be a tight Achilles tendon. Consult your doctor who may well ask an orthopaedic specialist or a paediatric physiotherapist to have a look at your child. Frequently, gentle stretching and physiotherapy is all that is required, and only about one per cent of children need further treatment for this.

If a child who used to be able to walk normally begins to walk on his or her toes, then you should seek medical advice. Sometimes this is a sign of tightness in the muscles that could result from a mild neurological problem from the time of birth, which should be assessed properly.

Overlapping toes

Many babies have toes that overlap. Gentle stretching will help the great majority to straighten out before the age of three. If the problem persists after this, then see your doctor. It is possible that surgery may be needed, but this is not urgent. The chief problem resulting from overlapping toes can be that it is difficult to find shoes that fit!

THE ARMS

Pulled elbows

This is a remarkably common phenomenon. It typically occurs when your child pulls against you when you are holding his or her hand, if you swing the child around by the arms, or if you suddenly pull on the arm. One of the bones in the elbow joint temporarily comes out of place, and whilst it usually returns to normal straight away, one of the ligaments can be trapped between the bones and this leaves the child reluctant or unable to use the arm. Typically, your child will hold the arm slightly bent, with the palm facing downwards.

Every doctor is taught a simple manoeuvre that will 'unpull' the elbow quickly and relatively painlessly, so do seek help right away (though occasionally the joint sorts itself out as you are on your way to the casualty unit, and you arrive there to find your child is happy, healthy, and pain free!).

Painful wrists

If your child has a fall and appears to sprain his or her wrist, then do see a doctor about it. There is a high possibility that there will actually be a minor green-stick fracture. These are certainly much more common than sprains, and can be caused by relatively minor injuries. So, if in doubt about any wrist injury, please do see a doctor.

BACK PAIN

Whilst the back is one of the great design faults of the human body, and whilst back pain is extremely common in adults, it is actually very unusual for young children to suffer back pain. So if your child complains of a bad back, then you really ought to see a doctor. If your child seems to be passing more urine than normal, it is possible that the pain is coming from a urinary tract infection, so it would be worth taking a urine specimen with you when you see the doctor.

OTHER JOINT PROBLEMS

Juvenile rheumatoid arthritis

Rheumatoid arthritis is sometimes known as Still's disease when it affects children. Approximately one child in 1,500 will develop this condition, so it is not common. It is twice as likely to affect girls as boys, and it is most likely to occur between the ages of one and three, and eight and twelve.

This condition may cause swelling and pain in one or two joints only, most typically the knee, the elbow or the ankle, though sometimes it seems to affect far more joints than this. Children with this condition may develop a fever and feel generally unwell. It is certainly a condition that requires medical investigation and management, and most children with juvenile rheumatoid arthritis will be admitted to hospital. Bed rest, anti-inflammatory drugs, and physiotherapy all have a place in management, and most sufferers will make a full recovery with no lasting ill effects.

Lyme disease

Lyme disease is transmitted by tick bites, and can cause pain and swelling in a joint, especially the knee, often coming on about three weeks after the original bite. The joints are often not visibly inflamed, and some children may just limp because they say their knee is uncomfortable. Lyme disease is frequently associated with a rash, and is dealt with further in the chapter on 'The child with a rash'. It can be quite difficult to diagnose, but if, for instance, you have been camping in the highlands of Scotland, and three weeks later your child develops a painful knee, then it is a very real possibility.

Septic arthritis and osteomyelitis

Septic arthritis is a bacterial infection of a joint, and osteomyelitis is a bacterial infection of a bone. Whilst both these conditions used to be fairly common, they are now rare. The chief symptoms are a high fever with swelling and very marked tenderness over the affected area.

Septic arthritis and osteomyelitis typically happen in children aged under three years, and are most likely to affect the elbow, hip or knee. Whilst established cases are easy and obvious to diagnose, the first sign may simply be swelling in a joint. This is never normal in children, so you should see a doctor right away. The earlier that septic arthritis is treated, the fewer the problems it causes in the long-term.

Treatment is with very high doses of antibiotics, typically given into a vein initially – which means hospital admission. On occasions, if the antibiotics do not seem to be working quickly enough, a general anaesthetic may have to be given so that the bone or joint can be drained surgically.

Section Four

Infectious Diseases

Disease	Incubation Period	Infectious Period	Restrictions/Exclusions	Notes
Chickenpox	2–3 weeks	Infectious up to 5 days before and not more than 5 days after appearance of spots	Exclusion for at least 5 days after spots first appear or until spots become dry	Infection confers long immunity. Second attacks are rare
Cold Sores	2–12 days	Virus can be present up to 7 weeks after recovery from lesion on lip. Usually spread by direct contact or saliva	None	Good personal hygiene can minimise transfer of infection
Conjunctivitis	24–72 hrs	Can be infectious while eye is inflamed. Spread by contact, sharing flannels, etc.	Exclusion not usually necessary after medical treatment/advice	Good personal hygiene can minimise transfer of infection
Fifth Disease	4–20 days	Infectious before onset of rash but probably not after rash appears	Exclusion until clinically well	Rash has 'slapped face' appearance followed a day or so later by a lace-like rash on body
Glandular Fever	4–6 weeks	The virus may be carried by the affected person for a year or more after the illness. Transmission is via saliva, usually kissing	Exclusion until clinically well	
Hand, Foot & Mouth	3–5 days	Infectious during period of illness	Exclusion until clinically well	
Hepatitis A	15–50 days	The virus is spread from the faeces of an affected person to the mouth of another. The infectious period is during the last half of the incubation period, and for up to a week after the jaundice appears	Exclusion until one week after the jaundice appears plus clinically well	Scrupulous hygiene needed after going to lavatory
Impetigo	4–10 days	Infectious usually until the lesions have healed. The bacteria are usually spread by pus on fingers	Exclusion for 48 hours after treatment started unless lesions can be covered	Personal hygiene very important

Influenza	1–5 days	Infectious up to one week after onset	Exclusion until well	
Measles	7–18 days	Infectious from just before illness starts until 4 days after appearance of rash	Exclusion until well	Unimmunised persons can usually be vaccinated successfully if within 3 days of contact
Meningitis	Varies	according to cause (see section on Meningitis, p 103)		
Mumps	12–25 days	Infectious from one week before to one week after onset of facial swelling	Exclusion until swelling has subsided	
Rubella	14–23 days	Infectious for about 1 week before and at least 4 days after onset of rash	Exclusion for 7 days after onset of rash	Pregnant women should be made aware of this diagnosis
Scabies	2–6 weeks (1–4 days if previously infected)	Infectious until treated. Mites are transferred during skin-to-skin contact and via recently infected underclothes or bed linen	Exclusion until the day after treatment	The mites make tiny burrows in the skin which itch intensely, especially at night. Sites include between fingers, wrists, elbows, etc.
Scaret Fever or Scarlatina	1–3 days	Usually spread by direct contact. Infectious until treated with appropriate antibiotic for 48 hours	Exclusion until 48 hours after treatment	
Whooping Cough	7–10 days	Infectious from onset until about 3 weeks later (or 5 days if treated with appropriate antibiotic)	Exclusion for 3 weeks from onset. If treated with antibiotic can return when clinically well	During an outbreak, children under five years should not be admitted to school unless known to be immunised

Section Five

A Guide to Children's Medicines

Many of the conditions that this book has looked at need little treatment other than a cuddle, and perhaps some paracetamol. Nevertheless there are going to be occasions when your child will need medication, and whilst no parent enjoys using medicines, you really do need to understand about the commonest treatments, how they work, what side effects they may have, and so on. You may be the world's most caring parent, being meticulous about diet, hygiene, or keeping your children warm, but the simple fact is that all children do become ill with problems such as coughs, colds, fevers, or earache. On these occasions parents really need to know something about the medicines their child may be taking. How should they be stored? Should the full course be completed? How does the medicine work, and what side effects does it have?

No single chapter is going to be able to answer every question about every possible medicine. Such a task would take numerous books. As just a simple example, in one of the standard reference guides to prescribing for family doctors, known as MIMS, there are currently listed ninety-nine different antibiotics. Whilst some of these are the same drug under different names and manufactured by different companies, there are still a quite remarkably large number of entirely different available drugs.

This section can just give you an outline guide to the different groups of drugs used for children, and answer the most commonly asked questions about the most commonly used drugs. If you still have questions then do ask your family doctor or pharmacist. He or she should always be able to provide full information about any drug that your child might need.

ANTIBIOTICS

There are two main groups of antibiotics used in childhood. Penicillins, and non-penicillin antibiotics. If your child is allergic to the penicillins then the alternative group will be chosen – and these also have their own particular uses.

Examples

Penicillins – Amoxycillin, Amoxil, Augmentin, Penbritin, etc.

Other antibiotics – Ceporex, Distaclor, Erythromycin, Erythroped, Klaricid, Trimethoprim, etc.

What they do

Destroy the bacteria that can cause many childhood infections – such as many infections of the ear, chest, urine, and some throat infections. However they are useless against viruses, which cause most colds and sore throats.

Formulations

For children these are usually given as liquid medicines, though some are available as drops (useful for small babies), or pleasant-flavoured 'chew-tabs' or tablets.

Should the course be finished?

Usually your child will need to take a full five- or seven-day course. Do not stop when your child feels better or there is a real risk of the bacteria developing resistance so that the drug will be less effective next time. Some bottles contain more medicine than will be needed, so do check with your doctor as the prescription is written.

Side effects

Most antibiotics can cause rashes or diarrhoea. However, most rashes in children on antibiotics are probably not true allergies but are caused by the original infection. Do show your doctor or practice nurse the rash – rather than risking an unnecessary labelling of an allergy that doesn't exist.

Hints and tips

- Most antibiotics should be shaken well and stored in the fridge. Check on the label.
- Never give them to other children without checking with the doctor – however similar the symptoms might be.
- If your child won't take a particular flavour, do tell your doctor. An identical drug with a different flavour may be available.

PAIN KILLERS

Examples

The most common pain killer used for children is paracetamol. This is marketed as Calpol, Disprol or Panadol – and also comes in numerous other forms, including drops, which may be beneficial for very young infants. Aspirin is not safe for children aged under twelve. The chief alternative to paracetamol is ibuprofen. Alternative brands include Junifen, Brufen and Nurofen.

What they do

As well as easing pain, these drugs also help if your child has a fever, lowering the temperature back towards normal. Ibuprofen is also an anti-inflammatory drug, and recent studies have shown that it is at least as effective and as well tolerated as paracetamol in helping to lower a raised temperature.

Formulations

Mainly as syrups, and best chosen in the sugar-free form. Also available as suppositories for children who might be vomiting – but seek medical advice first.

Should the course be finished?

No. These drugs should only be given for as long as they are needed. In other words, carry on for as long as your child has a temperature or is in pain.

Side effects

Remarkably safe, provided the specified dose is not exceeded. Ibuprofen is not advised in children with asthma as it is thought that it can worsen wheezing. Do follow the instructions on the pack very closely.

Hints and tips

- All brands of paracetamol are as effective as any other brand. Choose the cheapest formulation that has a flavour which your child will take. Despite all the hype, the expensive brand names are no more effective than the cheaper alternatives, and carry no other important ingredients other than flavourings.

- Avoid drugs which combine a pain killer with some other preparation – such as cough linctus or anti-histamine. If the drug upsets your child you won't know which constituent was to blame.

ANTI-HISTAMINES

Examples

Piriton, Triludan, Dimotane, Clarityn, Phenergan, Optimine, Vallergan.

What they do

These drugs chiefly block the effects of histamine, which is a chemical released when the body comes into contact with something it is allergic to. They also have a use in relieving stuffy blocked noses, easing itching, and occasionally as mild sedatives.

Formulations

For children all these drugs come as pleasant-tasting medicines. However, do follow the instructions closely. Many have strict minimum age restrictions, and some of these have changed recently. Phenergan, for instance, has long been used in children but is no longer licensed for use in children under the age of two years.

Should the course be finished?

In general anti-histamines are simply used to treat symptoms, and so there is strictly speaking no need to take a full course. However if your child is being given anti-histamines for a condition such as hayfever the treatment will need to be taken for as long as the hayfever season lasts. Unlike antibiotics, there is no risk involved in stopping a course early, but the symptoms may return.

Side effects

Many of these drugs can cause sedation and sleepiness. Ask your doctor or pharmacist for advice if this could be a problem. Some – such as Triludan – are much less sedative than others, but mild sedation may be a useful thing in dealing with a child who is suffering with itching at bedtime.

Hints and tips

- Most so-called 'cold cures' are combinations of antihistamines with other drugs. Drug combinations are generally not a good idea and have a risk of causing more side effects.
- Do not use these drugs just to make your child sleep at night. They rarely work, and can cause daytime hangover and irritability.

COUGH MEDICINES

Examples

Simple Linctus BP, Benylin, Tixylix, Actifed Linctus.

What they do

These drugs are intended to soothe coughing, and are often combined with anti-histamines to ease congestion of the nose. However there is little good evidence that they work. These notes are intended for parents who are still keen to use cough medicines. Almost no cough medicines are available on prescription, and if you want to use them you will need to purchase them. Despite their selling in millions of bottles, the British National Formulary – the U.K.'s most authoritative guide to prescribing – says of them: 'The drawbacks of prescribing cough suppressants are rarely outweighed by the benefits of treatment, and only occasionally are they useful.'

Formulations

All children's preparations come as syrups.

Should the course be finished?

No. They are not intended to cure, just to soothe. Stop when the cough is better.

Side effects

Those which include anti-histamines can cause sleepiness. Many can cause constipation. Occasionally they can cause confusion.

Hints and tips

- Save your money. Soothing warm drinks – such as Ribena, or honey and lemon mixtures can be just as effective at easing coughing, especially if paracetamol is given as well.

- If you are keen to give a cough medicine, then Simple Linctus Paediatric BP will be available at your pharmacist's and is very cheap indeed.
- Never use adult cough medicines for small children.

DECONGESTANTS

Examples

Oral Medicines include Sudafed, Actifed.

Nasal preparations (drops and sprays) include Otrivine, Ephedrine, Afrazine, Fenox.

What they do

These drugs are designed to reduce nasal congestion – for instance in colds or hayfever.

Formulations

Liquid medicines, nose drops, sprays.

Should the course be finished?

No. These drugs are simply designed to ease symptoms. Stopping treatment early will do no harm.

Side effects

The decongestant medicines can almost all cause drowsiness, or occasionally the opposite – sleeplessness. The nasal preparations should never be used for more than seven days.

They are of limited value, and can cause a rebound problem in which as the treatment wears off the symptoms seem to get worse, which may tempt you to use more and more treatment. The longer treatment is used, the worse this problem becomes.

Hints and tips

- Simple anti-histamines are almost always as good as this group of drugs, and are likely to be much cheaper. The British National Formulary (the doctors' bible on modern medication) says that decongestants are all 'of doubtful value'.
- You should never be tempted to use adult medicines for children.
- Sniffing warm moist air can be every bit as effective as any other decongestants and has far fewer side effects. Some people find that inhalations such as Vick, Karvol, or menthol can make this even more effective.

ASTHMA TREATMENTS

Asthma is becoming increasingly common, with approximately one child in eight having the condition. There are two main groups of treatment – preventers and relievers. I will deal with these separately.

ASTHMA RELIEVERS

Examples

Ventolin, Salbutamol, Bricanyl, Aerolin, Pulmadil, Salamol, Terbutaline.

What they do

These drugs relieve spasms in the bronchi (the airways in the lungs). They generally work remarkably quickly. They should be used if your child is wheezy, or occasionally may be recommended before exercise. Some doctors may advise you to use a dose of a reliever before giving a preventer drug. The logic behind this is that any wheeze will be cleared which then allows the preventer to work more effectively.

Incidentally, babies often do not respond to the standard asthma treatments, and a drug called Atrovent (ipratropium bromide) may be offered instead until the baby is older.

Formulations

These may be given as liquid medicines, or as various types of inhaler device. (See next section.) One reliever – Slo-Phyllin – comes as a capsule full of granules which can be sprinkled on jam or yogurt.

Should the course be finished?

Unless your doctor or nurse advises you specifically, these drugs are mainly designed to ease symptoms. Using them regularly is nowhere near as important as it is with the preventer drugs.

Side effects

The main side effect is a fine tremor, or shake. This is much less likely to occur with inhaled drugs where the dose of drugs used is very much smaller. Some parents find that these treatments seem to 'wind up' their children. If you think this may be happening, talk to your doctor and possibly experiment with an alternative preparation.

ASTHMA PREVENTERS

Examples

Becotide, Pulmicort, Aerobec, Beclazone, Flixotide, Beclamethazone, Intal.

What they do

These drugs are known as anti-inflammatories. They work by damping down the inflammation of the lining of the airways in the lung which appears to be the cause of most asthma. Preventing wheeze and cough occurring is far more important than treating wheezing after it has started. For the great majority of asthmatic children these are absolutely essential. There is some evidence that the use of relievers alone can actually worsen the inflammation in the bronchi. For all except children who only wheeze rarely, preventer drugs are vitally important.

Formulations

These drugs all come as inhalers. Some are given through large transparent plastic devices called large volume spacers (Volumatic or Nebuhaler). Others can be given by dry powder inhalers. Your doctor or nurse should be able to go through the options with you to find a treatment that your child is happy to use.

Should the course be finished?

It is absolutely essential that these treatments are used regularly – usually twice every day, until you are advised otherwise. They are almost useless if you simply use them when you think they are needed. Regular use can make a fantastic difference to the severity of the asthma, and how well your child feels and sleeps.

Side effects

These drugs are almost all tiny doses of steroids (with the exception of Intal), and in general these have very few side effects provided they are used in the correct doses. They can occasionally cause an infection of thrush in the mouth. Intal (dysodium cromoglycate) is virtually free of side effects and is often used as a first-line preventative treatment, but it is not always effective.

Hints and tips

- If your child is struggling with any one particular inhaler device, do let your doctor or nurse know. There may be an alternative design which will suit much better.
- The chief sign that childhood asthma is not being well enough controlled is usually cough, not wheeze.
- If your child goes to playgroup or has started school, do ensure that someone knows that he or she has asthma and has a supply of a reliever drug to use in an emergency.
- Electric nebulisers can seem an easy and effective way of giving treatment, but they are not prescribable on the NHS, and in infants there is evidence that some of the therapies that help older children and adults can cause

irritation to the lining of the bronchi and actually make wheezing worse.

ECZEMA TREATMENTS

Examples

There are two main groups of treatment for eczema, which is a condition in which the skin becomes excessively dry and inflamed.

Emollients: Emulsiderm, Oilatum, Emulsifying Ointment, Balneum, Unguentum Merck.

Steroid Creams: Hydrocortisone, Eumovate, Betnovate, Propaderm.

There are of course many other approaches to eczema, but this section can only cover commonly used medication.

What they do

Emollients help to soften and moisturise the skin.

Anti-inflammatory (steroid) creams deal with the underlying inflammation.

Formulations

Emollients come as creams, lotions, and bath oils. Adding a couple of capfuls to bath water can be a very effective way of softening the skin.

The steroids mainly come as creams and ointments. Creams are generally less greasy than ointments, but ointments are better for long-term very dry scaly rashes.

Should the course be finished?

Use the shortest course of the lowest strength of steroid cream or ointment that clears the rash effectively (your doctor will advise on this), but continue emollients even after the skin appears better. These will help to prevent flare-ups and are entirely safe.

Side effects

Topical steroids can cause thinning of the skin if too high a dose is used for too long. They are wonderfully effective drugs if used in the right dose for the right length of time. Do discuss this with your doctor.

Hints and tips

- Emollients are entirely safe, and can be used by any member of the family. It is quite safe to share bath water, for instance, if emollients have been added. Steroid creams should never be used on another child without medical advice.
- Emollients do make children – and baths – very slippery, so take care!

The National Eczema Society provides excellent leaflets on treatments in eczema. Write to Tavistock House North, London WC1H 9SR.

STEROIDS

Steroids – properly known as corticosteroids – are extremely powerful drugs which can be remarkably effective in all manner of medical conditions. If not used with care, however, they can be hazardous. The risks do cause many parents to panic and to be extremely reluctant to allow their children to be given such treatments. In fact, in conditions like asthma the appropriate use of steroids can be life-saving, and avoiding them can be extremely hazardous. It is therefore important that parents understand these drugs.

Examples and formulations

Lung inhalers: include Becotide, Becloforte, Pulmicort, Aerobec, Beclamethasone, Flixotide.

Nasal Inhalers: include Beconase, Flixonase, Rhinacort, Syntaris.

Tablets: Prednisolone, Prednesol, Beclamethasone, Cortisone.

In addition, they are available in eye drops, ointments and creams.

How they work

Steroids occur naturally in the body. They are produced by the adrenal gland, and their chief function is reducing inflammation. This is why they are so useful in conditions such as asthma where persistent inflammation is a major problem, in particular in disorders where the body's immune system appears to be faulty in some way. This can include conditions like asthma, hayfever, some blood disorders, inflammation of the eyes, the skin, or the bowel, and rheumatoid arthritis.

Should the course be finished?

It is essential that you know from your doctor whether any steroid treatment is supposed to be a short course, or for more prolonged treatment. In most cases in children these drugs will be used in an inhaled form. These should be used on a regular continual basis. However, doctors will always aim to use steroids that are given by mouth in the lowest possible dose for the shortest length of time. But do not stop treatment without checking with your doctor first.

Side effects

There is a risk that long-term oral steroids (that is steroids given by mouth) can affect a child's growth. This is the chief reason that courses will be kept short. You may find these drugs so remarkably effective in reducing your child's symptoms that you wonder why they cannot be continued. Oral steroids taken for too long can also cause muscle wasting, thinning of the skin, fluid retention, weight gain, reduced ability to fight infection, and so on. These are tremendously powerful drugs, with great benefits, but significant risks. Your doctor should discuss the pros and cons of this form of treatment with you. Inhaled steroids have far fewer problems. Recent evidence suggests that inhaled steroids are very much safer when it comes to interfering with growth. It seems likely that Flixotide and Flixonase may be the safest, but this only seems to apply if high dosages are being used. Do discuss this with your doctor.

Hints and tips

- There are many different types of inhaled steroids available. Some are much easier to administer than others. If you have problems with one, talk to your doctor.
- Never stop steroid treatments without seeking medical advice first.

- Inhaled steroids may cause thrush in the mouth. Large volume spacer devices make this much less likely.

LONG-TERM MEDICATIONS

Children with chronic (long-term) medical problems such as epilepsy or diabetes will almost certainly need to be on medication all the time. Examples of the types of drug that are involved include insulin injections for diabetic children, and drugs like Epilim, sodium valproate, phenytoin, or Tegretol in epilepsy.

With these long-term medications it is essential that parents should understand the drugs in some detail. If your child needs continual drugs, can you answer the following questions?

1. How often should the drug be given?
2. What should you do if your child misses a dose?
3. What should you do if your child vomits, or is otherwise unwell?
4. What are the side effects?
5. Should it be taken with food, or on an empty stomach?

If you are certain of the answer to all the above, then all is well. If not, then why not make a copy of this list and take it to the doctor next time you attend. Caring for a child with a long-term medical problem has to be a partnership between parents and doctor, and doctors should be more than happy to discuss these types of problem with you. It really is important that parents feel confident and able to talk to their doctor. If your doctor is not happy to discuss these matters with you, then it might be worth talking to another of the partners if it is a group practice, or even transferring to a different practice if this is practicable.

These days patients do not have to give any reason for changing doctors. A good relationship between parent and doctor is an essential part of childcare, and there is little point in persevering with a relationship that has broken down. If you want more detail, then most long-term medical problems have self-help groups which can provide you with leaflets and booklets on all forms of medication.

GENERAL ADVICE

- Most medicines are available in sugar-free forms. Choose these whenever possible.
- If in doubt ask. That is precisely what your doctor or pharmacist is there for.
- If you have concerns about any medication, do not just stop giving it. Seek medical advice first.
- Do not always expect to receive a prescription at the end of every consultation. The great majority of childhood problems will get better without drugs. If your doctor doesn't prescribe, it doesn't mean that he or she does not believe you or take you seriously.
- With small babies, medicine spoons can be difficult to use. You and the baby are likely to end up sticky and irritable! Ask your pharmacist for a dosage syringe which makes giving medicine much easier.
- Indeed, most medicine spoons are a disastrous example of bad design. They have to be filled to the brim, which means that it is almost inevitable you will spill some. Why not obtain either a dosage syringe, or a well designed measuring aid, for any child?
- Never give any child medication that was prescribed for someone else.

QUESTIONS TO ASK YOUR DOCTOR ABOUT ANY PRESCRIBED MEDICATION

- How long is the course?
- Do I stop giving it when my child seems better?
- When should I give it?
- Does it have to be given with food?
- How should it be stored?
- Is it safe to give paracetamol with this if it is needed?
- What side effects might I expect?
- Do I need to bring my child back for a check-up after treatment?

GIVING MEDICINES TO CHILDREN

Giving medicine to a child can be a real battle, even when medicines have been formulated to taste good. Countless parents have struggled with a screaming toddler who clamps his lips together in a desperate attempt to avoid being given medication. Trying to slip a spoon between gritted gums whilst your child is shaking his head from side to side can test the patience of any parent – particularly when you yourself end up covered in a spoonful of sticky antibiotic.

So how can you make giving medicines less of a stressful chore? Perhaps the most useful new gadget that really helps parents has been the arrival of the oral dosage syringe. These syringes are provided automatically by the pharmacist if the dose of the medicine is less than a full 5ml – the average spoonful. They can also be purchased, or your doctor may prescribe them. They are provided with an adapter that fits into the top of the medicine bottle, and the syringes are marked in 0.5ml divisions from one to 5ml if you need to give dosages of less than 5ml.

When giving medicines using these syringes, make sure your child is sitting up. Trying to give medicines to a child who is lying down can be dangerous, as the child may inhale rather than swallow. Aim into the side of the mouth, and push the plunger down very slowly. Do *not* squirt the medicine at high speed into the back of your child's throat, or gagging will almost certainly result.

If you are using a normal 5ml medicine spoon, do ensure that it is full – if a full 5ml dose is what the label instructs. Unfortunately the design of many of the spoons provided free with many medicines is completely hopeless. The dose is only accurate when the spoon is full, but it is almost impossible to give a full spoon without spilling it. There are a number of commercially available spoons with a sensible lip to them, so if you don't use a dosage syringe, consider investing in one of these.

How easy it is to give medication will depend on many factors, in particular the age of your child. However, your own attitude can make a tremendous difference. If you give the impression that a medicine is unpleasant, then your child is bound to react unfavourably. It is all a bit like going to the dentist. Many parents effectively teach their children to be frightened of the dentist. They use phrases like 'be brave', or 'if you're good I'll buy you some sweets' – phrases that you would never use about a trip to the park. Children are not stupid. If bribery is needed, they will assume the experience is bound to be unpleasant. So try to keep a matter-of-fact approach, and if you are bad at taking medicines, try to disguise this.

Some parents find it easier to transfer a spoonful of medicine into a small cup, and then give it a little at a time. This way, if any is spat out it can be collected and regiven. However, it isn't really wise to put medicine into a large volume of drink as it may not all be taken. Instead, if necessary have a drink on offer to give as soon as the medicine is finished.

If no amount of persuasion will allow you to give your toddler so much as a drop of medicine, you may need help. One of you can hold the child with his or her arms restrained, whilst the other has the medicine ready to give. But whatever you do, don't deceive your child by pretending the medicine is something it isn't. This may work for one dose, but you will have an even bigger battle on your hands next time. And if your child really does find a particular medicine completely unpalatable, have a word with your doctor to see if there is an alternative preparation with a more pleasant taste.

Ear drops

When giving ear drops, lie your child on one side, or else tip the head away from the side that you want to put the drops. Then hold the dropper close to the ear, and gently squeeze the rubber bulb so that the drops are released into the ear canal. It is then best to leave the child in this position for a couple of minutes, and repeat this on the other side if necessary.

Nose drops

In babies, it is best to lie your baby across your knee with the neck resting on your thigh. Gently support the head with one hand, put the dropper inside the nostril and insert the necessary number of drops, then repeat this in the other nostril. In older children, it is best if your child blows his or her nose first. Then he or she should lie down looking upwards, with the neck resting on a bunched-up pillow and the head tilted backwards, and in this position it is easy to insert the drops. Wait a minute or so before letting your child get up again.

Eye drops

It is usually best to have help when trying to put eye drops into young children, unless they are remarkably co-operative. One of you should hold the head steady, and the other holds the dropper in one hand, resting the hand against the child's forehead. Now with the index finger of the other hand gently pull the lower eyelids downwards. Then gently squeeze the drops into the area between the eye and the lower eyelid. Do not touch the eye with the dropper. If you are using an eye ointment, use a similar technique, again rolling the lower lid downwards, and squeeze a small amount of the ointment along the inside of the eyelid – just like squeezing toothpaste onto a toothbrush. Your child will then blink, and the blinking spreads the ointment over the whole surface of the eye.

Medicine labels

Whilst in the past, medicine labels contained remarkably little information other than the bare words 'To be taken as directed', modern labels give a great deal of information. Always read these labels carefully. Check how the medicine should be stored. Should it be kept cool, or even in the fridge? Should it be shaken before use? Are other medications safe if taken at the same time? Should the course be completed? What side effects are there? Many medications containing anti-histamines and which are formulated for small children contain the advice, 'Avoid driving or using heavy machinery'. Some advice does seem rather unnecessary, but in general the more information you have, the better. Indeed, if you are in doubt about any aspect of using the medication, ask the pharmacist or your doctor.

A HOME MEDICINE CHEST

There are a huge number of medicines advertised for treating family illnesses. Parents can quite justifiably feel confused when faced with the selection advertised so colourfully in the parenting press, or on sale at their local pharmacy.

So, when you need to treat your child at home for a minor illness such as a sore throat, tummy upset, cough, or cold, how on earth do you begin to know what is the best medicine to use? The next box lists the contents that I would recommend you keep in a home medicine chest for treating children's illnesses. I suspect that it will surprise you. You may think it is a short list. However, these are the only 'over-the-counter' medicines that I have ever used for my own children throughout their entire childhood. If my children didn't need more than this, I doubt if yours do either. You simply don't need large numbers of drugs. Obviously, if your child has some long-term medical problem such as asthma or eczema you will also need the relevant drugs that your G.P. prescribes or advises. This list here is aimed at the average family, and should cover most important everyday medical needs.

A BASIC HOME MEDICINE CHEST

- Paracetamol medicine (such as Calpol or Disprol)
- Paracetamol tablets for older children and adults
- Rehydration sachets for diarrhoea (such as Rehidrat or Dioralyte)
- Calamine lotion for itching rashes or bites
- For babies: cream to prevent nappy rash, such as zinc and castor oil
- An anti-histamine, such as Piriton, can be helpful for any form of itch or allergy

Whilst paracetamol is generally the most commonly prescribed and used pain killer for use in children, there is no doubt that ibuprofen can also be extremely effective and may suit some children better. Ibuprofen is known as an anti-inflammatory analgesic. This means that as well as relieving pain, it helps to damp down inflammation. It is generally best avoided in children with asthma, but this is detailed fully in the guide to children's medicines included in this book, along with the use of re-hydration sachets.

Do-s and don't-s for over-the-counter medication

Despite the shortness of my recommended list of medication, I do realise that many parents feel that they want or need to purchase other treatments such as cough medicines. When you are purchasing medicines, do make sure that the pharmacist knows the age of your child, as there are usually different formulations for different ages.

There are also some simple rules for using medication that you should always try to follow:

- Make sure that you know exactly what the dose is, and how often it should be given. And do make sure that you use the spoon provided. Most doses are measured in 5ml spoons. If you use a teaspoon, you may be giving a smaller dose than is recommended or needed. Measuring syringes, available from all pharmacists, are actually much more accurate to use.

- Ask if the medicine has any side effects. Some antihistamines and cough medicines can make children sleepy. You will worry less if you know what to expect.
- Check the expiry date on any medicines in your medicine cabinet, and throw away any that are out of date.
- Make sure that any medicines that you keep in the house are firmly locked away. Don't simply leave them on a shelf, or in an unlocked cupboard where your child might be able to get hold of them. Medication may come in child-proof bottles, but many children find these easier to open than do adults!
- If you know that your child is allergic to specific food or colouring additives, do ask for brands of medicine which don't contain colouring or ingredients to which he or she might react.
- Don't offer your children sweets or other bribes as a reward for taking their medicines, or they quickly get the idea that any medicine is going to be unpleasant. In fact, most medicines designed for children nowadays have a genuinely pleasant flavour.

Section Six

Practical Techniques

HOW TO TAKE YOUR CHILD'S TEMPERATURE

Babies

With small babies the most accurate way of taking the temperature is by inserting a thermometer in the rectum. However, I really do believe that this is only wise if you have been carefully taught this technique by a doctor or nurse and if you genuinely feel confident and safe in doing this. Using a thermometer – either electronic or mercury – in the armpit can give a good idea of your baby's temperature and is much safer. However, temperatures recorded in this way give a reading which is generally about one degree Fahrenheit lower than in the mouth. Strip thermometers, such as Feverscan, which are used on the forehead have the virtue of being very safe and very hygienic, although they are not terribly accurate and can only really give a rough guide to whether your baby has a temperature or not. To be honest that is often all that you need to know. It is far more important to be able to judge how ill your child is, rather than to be able to take a scientifically accurate and very precise recording of the temperature.

The older child

For older children, the most accurate way of taking the temperature is by using a thermometer under the tongue. This should ideally be left in place for at least a full minute. If you take the temperature in the armpit, leave the thermometer in place for at least three minutes. Forehead fever strips are also frequently quite accurate enough for older children, and even adults, though no one can pretend they are as accurate as the more traditional forms of thermometer.

EMERGENCY RESUSCITATION FOR PARENTS

This section aims to give quick and clear guidance to the vitally important techniques required if your child stops breathing for any reason. Unlike the rest of the book, I have not explained in detail what the rationale and explanation for everything is. In an emergency, you just have to get on and do it. Now!

However, I would strongly advise all parents to get real expertise in first aid. Contact your local St John's Ambulance Brigade, or find out if there are suitable local evening classes. Every adult should understand first aid. You really can save a life.

Babies aged under twelve months

- If someone is with you make sure they send for a 999 ambulance now. If you are alone, go through the cycle of artificial respiration twice and then urgently call yourself before you start again
- Straighten your baby's neck, lift the jaw very slightly, and cover the baby's nose and mouth with your mouth
- Blow just hard enough to move your baby's chest up and down, and keep this going at a rate of about one breath every three seconds. (An easy way to count seconds is to say '121, 122, 123 . . .')
- After each breath, briefly lift your mouth away from your baby's mouth, to let the air escape from the baby's mouth before you repeat the cycle
- Keep doing this until either your baby starts breathing spontaneously, or an ambulance arrives

Children aged over one year

- Tilt your child's head back slightly, and lift the jaw so that it is slightly lifted forwards
- Squeeze the child's nose, so that air cannot pass through it
- Put your mouth over your child's, and blow in so as to make the chest rise. Incidentally, don't be too aggressive. You may only have to breathe quite gently
- Allow air to escape from your child's mouth between each breath
- Keep going at a rate of about one breath every four seconds
- Make sure that someone sends for an ambulance right away. If you are alone try not to panic, but do the whole cycle of artificial respiration twice, then send for a 999 ambulance. Then return to your child until either breathing starts spontaneously, or an ambulance arrives

Section Seven

Useful Organisations

The organisations listed here can all provide excellent and valuable help for parents. Most of them are run on tight budgets, so please enclose return postage when contacting them.

Accidents
Child Accident Prevention Trust
28 Portland Place
London W1N 4DE

Asthma
National Asthma Campaign
300 Upper Street
Islington
London N1 2XX

Crying
Serene (formerly Cry-Sis)
BM Cry-sis
London WC1N 3XX

Cystic fibrosis
The Cystic Fibrosis Trust
Alexandra House
5 Blyth Rd
Bromley
Kent BR1 3RS

Diabetes
The British Diabetic Association
10 Queen Anne Street
London W1M 0BD
Tel: 0171 323 1531
Careline: 0171 636 6112

Eating problems (such as Anorexia or Bulimia)
Eating Disorders Association
Sackville Place
44 Magdalen Street
Norwich NR3 1JU

Eczema
National Eczema Society
163 Eversholt Street
London NW1 1BU

Epilepsy
British Epilepsy
Association
Anstey House
40 Hanover Square
Leeds LS3 1BE
Freephone Helpline:
0800 30 90 30

First Aid
St John's Ambulance
National Headquarters
1 Grosvenor Crescent
London SW1X 7EF

Hyperactivity
The Hyperactive Children's
Support Group
71 Whyke Lane
Chichester
West Sussex PO19 2LD

Migraine
The Migraine Trust
45 Great Ormond Street
London WC1N 3HZ

Index of Symptoms

Abdominal Pain: 68, 147–154
Anus, pain: 135–6, 140–1, 185
Anus, itching: 145, 184–186
Back pain: 292–293
Bedwetting: 162–166
Bites: 197–198
Bladder control: 163–164
Blood in stools: 140–142
Bottom, itchy: 184–185
Bow legs: 284
Catarrh: 108
Chills: 24, 63
Choking: 57–59
Cold sores: 212–213
Colds: 61–67
Conjunctivitis – 262–266
Conjunctivitis, allergic: 186, 267–8
Constipation: 134–139
Convulsions: 274–281
Cough: 39–49
Croup: 43, 46
Crying: 32–38
Dandruff: 201, 21 0
Deafness: 95–91
Dehydration: 123, 129
Depression: 32
Diarrhoea: 126–133
Dirt eating: 145
Discharge from ear: 77, 82–84
Dribbling urine: 166
Earache: 63, 73–81
Eye – red: 260–268
Eye, cloudy: 270–271
Eyelids, swollen: 271–272
Eyes, itching: 186
Faints: 281–282
Fatty Stools: 146
Feet, curved: 290
Feet, flat: 290
Fever: 21–26
Fits: 274–281
Flea bites: 197–298
Foreign body, inhaled: 46
Foreign body (nose): 108
Foreskin – problems: 172–3
Fractures: 283–284
Gastro-enteritis: 122, 127–131
Genitals – injury: 174 (boys)
Genitals – injury: 179 (girls)
Glands in neck: 93–94
Groin – swelling: 179–181
Hayfever: 108, 186, 240–245
Headache: 96–104
Hearing Problems: 85–91
Herpes Simplex (mouth ulcers): 112
Herpes Simplex: 212–3
Hip problems: 287–288
Hyperactivity: 254–256
Inhaled foreign body: 57
Itching: 182–188
Jaw joint pain: 74, 78
Knees, painful: 286
Knock knee: 285
Labia – problems with: 178–179
Legs, painful: 285–286
Limping: 286–287
Meningitis: 92, 98–9, **103–4**, 190
Mouth breathing: 108–109

Mouth ulcers: 112
Nappy Rash: 231–234
Nasal septum-displaced: 107
Nasal congestion: 107–108
Neck, swollen: 93–94
Neck, stiff: 92–93
Neck, painful: 92–93
Nose bleeds: 105–107
Nose, runny: 61
Nose, blocked: 61, 66
Pain: 27–31
Penis – problems: 174
Perforated ear drum: 76
Pigeon Toes: 288–289
Posseting: 120
Projectile vomiting: 121
Rashes: 189–230
Rashes, diagnosing: 191–194
Redcurrant jelly stool: 141, 153
Scalp, itching: 186–7
Sleep problems: 38
Sneezing: 110
Sniffing: 111
Snoring: 108–109
Soiling: 138
Sore Throat: 68–72
Speech problems – 85
Squint: 269–270
Stool, blood in motions: 140–142
Stool, abnormal colour: 142–144
Stools, abnormal: 140–146
Teething: 116–117
Testicle, undescended: 171–172
Throat, sore: 68–72
Toes, overlapping: 291
Toes, walking on: 291
Tongue tie: 113
Tonsillitis: 68–69
Tooth decay: 116–117
Tooth-damage to: 118
Toothache: 116
Travel sickness: 122
Tummy ache: 29, 147–149, 167
Urine discoloured: 160–162
Urine, frequency: 157
Urine, dribbling: 166
Urine, pain on passing: 155–157
Urine, cloudy: 162
Urine, offensive smell: 159
Vagina, foreign body: 178
Vaginal problems: 175–176
Vomiting: 64, 120–125
Vulva – problems with: 178–179
Watering eyes: 246–247
Wax in ear: 82
Wheeze: 51–60
Whooping Cough: 42, 49
Wind: 152
Wrist, painful: 292

Index

Abdominal Pain: 68, 147–154
Allergic Rhinitis: 108, 240–245
Allergic conjunctivitis: 246–247
Allergies: 195–196, 238–259
Anal fissure: 135–6, 140–1, 185
Analgesics: 303–305
Anaphylactic Shock: 257–259
Anti-histamines: 244, 305–306
Antibiotics: 13, 70, 302–303
Anus, itching: 145, 184–186
Anxiety: 158
Aphthous Ulcers: 112
Appendicitis: 150–1
Arthritis, septic: 294
Aspirin: 25
Asthma: 40–41, 51–60
Asthma, Medication: 309–313
Athlete's foot: 196–7, 210
Atopic families: 53, 202
Back pain: 292–293
Bedwetting: 162–166
Bites: 197–198
Bladder control: 163–164
Blepharitis: 263
Blood in stools: 140–142
Bottom, itchy: 184–185
Bow legs: 284
Brain tumour: 100
Bronchiectasis: 45
Bronchiolitis: 42, 52
Bronchitis: 41, 43
Calpol: 25
Carbon monoxide poisoning: 100
Cataract: 270
Catarrh: 108
Chickenpox: 198–200
Chills: 24, 63
Choking: 57–59
Co-ops (medical): 14
Coeliac Disease: 146
Cold sores: 212–213
Colds: 61–67
Colic: 151–152
Conjunctivitis: 262–266
Conjunctivitis, allergic: 186, 267–8
Constipation: 134–139
Convulsion – coping with: 280–1
Convulsion, febrile: 276–277
Convulsions: 274–281
Coryza: 61
Cough medicine: 306–308
Cough: 39–49
Coxsackie Virus: 229
Cradle Cap: 201
Croup: 43, 46
Cry-Sis: 36
Crying: 32–38
Cystic Fibrosis: 45, 133
Dandruff: 201, 210
Deafness: 95–91
Decongestants: 308–309
Dehydration: 123, 129
Dental caries: 116–117
Dental abscess: 118
Dentist: 119
Depression: 32

Dermatitis: 201
Diabetes: 158
Diarrhoea: 126–133
Digestion: 126
Dirt eating: 145
Discharge from ear: 77, 82–84
Doctors: 11–18
Dribbling urine: 166
Drug allergy: 196, 228
Drugs: 301–331
Ear drops: 321
Earache: 63, 73–81
Ears-examination of: 17
Echo Virus: 229
Eczema treatment: 313–314
Eczema: 185, 195–196, 200–205
Elbow, pulled: 292
Encephalitis: 217
Encopresis: 138
Enuresis: 162–166
Epididymitis: 174
Epiglottitis: 56, 64
Epilepsy: 278–281
Epistaxis: 105–107
Erythema Multiforme: 205–206
Erythema Nodosum: 206–207
Eustachian Tube congestion: 74, 78
Eye drops: 321
Eye – red: 260–268
Eye. anatomy: 260–262
Eye, cloudy: 270–271
Eyelids, swollen: 271–272
Eyes, itching: 186
Faints: 281–282
Fatty Stools: 146
Febrile convulsion: 23
Feet, curved: 290
Feet, flat: 290
Fever: 21–26
Fifth Disease: 207–208
Fits: 274–281
Flea bites: 197–298
Food allergy: 247–252
Food intolerance: 149, 252–256
Foreign body, inhaled: 46
Foreign body (nose): 108
Foreskin – problems: 172–3
Fractures: 283–284
Fungal infections: 196–7, 208–210
Gastro-enteritis: 122, 127–131
Genitals – injury: 174 (boys)
Genitals – injury: 179 (girls)
Geographical Tongue: 114
German Measles: 210–211
Glands in neck: 93–94
Glaucoma: 270
Glue ear: 86, 90
Grandparents: 4
Greenstick injuries: 284
Groin – swelling: 179–181
Grommets: 90
Hand, foot and mouth disease: 211–2
Hayfever: 108, 186, 240–245
Headache: 96–104
Health Visitors: 15, 35, 153
Hearing Problems: 85–91
Heimlich Manoeuvre: 58–9
Hernia: 180
Herpes Simplex (mouth ulcers): 112
Herpes Simplex: 212–3
Hip problems: 287–288
Hip, irritable: 287
Hirschsprung's disease: 135
Hives: 183
Hydrocoele: 173
Hyperactivity: 254–256
I.T.P.: 219–220
Immunisation: 42–43
Impetigo: 184, 213–214
Infantile Spasms: 278
Infection: 28
Infectious Diseases: 297–298
Inflammation: 28

Inhaled foreign body: 57
Intussusception: 141–2, 153
Iritis: 264
Itching: 182–188
Jaw joint pain: 74, 78
Kawasaki Disease: 214–5
Kidneys: 155–156
Knees, painful: 286
Knock knee: 285
Labia – problems with: 178–179
Lactose intolerance: 129–130, 253
Laxatives: 134, 136
Legs, painful: 285–286
Lice, head: 187–188
Limping: 286–287
Linctus: 48
Lungs: 40, 51
Lyme Disease: 215–216, 293–294
Lymph nodes: 93–4
Malabsorption: 146
Measles: 216–217
Meckel's Diverticulum: 141
Medication: 301–331
Medication, long term: 317–319
Medicine Chest, Home: 323–324
Meningitis: 92, 98–9, **103–4**, 190
Mesenteric adenitis: 68, 154
Migraine: 98, 101
Molluscum Contagiosum: 218
Mouth breathing: 108–109
Mouth ulcers: 112
Mycoplasma: 45
Nappy Rash: 231–234
Nasal allergies: 240–245
Nasal congestion: 107–108
Nasal septum-displaced: 107
Nebuliser: 44
Neck, swollen: 93–94
Neck, stiff: 92–93
Neck, painful: 92–93
Nose drops: 321
Nose bleeds: 105–107
Nose, runny: 61
Nose, blocked: 61, 66
Osgood-Schlatter's Disease: 286
Osteomyelitis: 294
Otitis Externa: 74, 77–8
Otitis Media: 74–76, 89
Pain killers: 303–305
Pain: 27–31
Paraphimosis: 172
Parvovirus: 207–208
Peak Flow Diary: 56
Penis – problems: 174
Perforated ear drum: 76, 89
Periodic Syndrome: 148–149
Perthe's Disease: 287
Pertussis: 42, 49
Petechiae: 218–220
Pica: 145
Pigeon Toes: 288–289
Pityriasis Rosea: 209, 220–221
Pneumonia: 42
Posseting: 120
Preventer inhaler: 56
Projectile vomiting: 121
Psoriasis: 221–2
Pyloric Stenosis: 120–121
Rashes: 189–230
Rashes, diagnosing: 191–194
Redcurrant jelly stool: 141, 153
Rehydration: 124, 130–132
Resuscitation: 330–331
Rheumatoid Arthritis: 293
Ringworm: 196–197, 208–210
Roseola Infantum: 222
Rubella: 87, 210–211
Scabies: 183–184, 223–225
Scalp, itching: 186–7
Scarlatina (Scarlet Fever): 225–226
Scrotum – problems: 173–174

Seborrhoeic Dermatitis: 226–227
Serene: 38
Shingles: 199–200
Sickle-cell anaemia: 208
Sinusitis: 99
Skin, structure & function: 191
Sleep problems: 38
Smoking: 49. 67, 81
Sneezing: 110
Sniffing: 111
Snoring: 108–109
Soiling: 138
Sore Throat: 68–72
Speech problems: 85
Sputum: 47
Squint: 269–270
Starving: 131
Steam: 44, 47, 66
Steroids: 314–317
Still's Disease: 293
Stool, blood in motions: 140–142
Stool-abnormal colour: 142–144
Stools, abnormal: 140–146
Strangulated hernia: 180
Stress: 158
Stye: 271
Swimming: 77, 84
Teething: 116–117
Telephone advice: 12
Temperature, taking: 329–330
Temperature-normal: 21
Tension headache: 97
Testicle, undescended: 171–172
Testicle, torsion: 174
Thermometers: 21–22
Threadworms: 144–145, 175
Throat, sore: 68–72
Throat-examination of: 18
Thrush: 232
Thyroid gland: 95
Ticks: 215–216
Toddler diarrhoea: 128
Toes, overlapping: 291
Toes, walking on: 291
Tongue tie: 113
Tonsillectomy: 70
Tonsillitis: 68–69
Tooth decay: 116–117
Tooth–damage to: 118
Toothache: 116
Travel sickness: 122
Tummy ache: 29, 147–149, 167
Ultrasound scan: 168
Upper Respiratory infection: 69
Urine discoloured: 160–162
Urine infection: 149, 156, 166–170
Urine, dribbling: 166
Urine, offensive smell: 159
Urine, pain on passing: 155–157
Urine, frequency: 157
Urine, cloudy: 162
Urticaria: 183, 227–229
Vagina, foreign body: 178
Vaginal problems: 175–176
Verrucae: 235–237
Virus infection: 61
Virus Rashes: 229–230
Volvulus: 154
Vomiting: 64
Vomiting: 120–125
Vulva – problems with: 178–179
Warts: 235–237
Watering eyes: 246–247
Wax in ear: 82
Wheeze: 51–60
Whooping Cough: 42, 49
Wind: 152
Wrist, painful: 292
Wry Neck: 92